W0228091

Essential Obstetrics

A guide to important principles
for nurses and laboratory technicians

Essential Obstetrics

for midwives and obstetric nurses

J. A. Chalmers

MD Edin FRCS Ed FRCOG
*Consultant Obstetrician and
Gynaecologist, Worcester Royal
Infirmary
Examiner, Royal College of
Obstetricians and Gynaecologists
and Central Midwives Board*

MTP

MEDICAL AND TECHNICAL PUBLISHING CO LTD
1973

Published by

MTP

Medical and Technical Publishing Co Ltd
St. Leonard's House, St. Leonardgate, Lancaster

Copyright © 1973, J. A. Chalmers

Softcover reprint of the hardcover 1st edition 1973

SBN 852 000 50 2

First published 1973

*No part of this book may be reproduced
in any form without permission from the
publishers except for the quotation of
brief passages for the purposes of review*

Books in the 'Essential knowledge' series for nurses:

Essential Anatomy
Essential Medicine
Essential Physics, Chemistry and Biology
**Essential Biochemistry, Endocrinology and
Nutrition**
Essential Diagnostic Tests
Essential Physiology

ISBN-13: 978-0-85200-050-2   e-ISBN-13: 978-94-010-2351-1
DOI: 10.1007/ 978-94-010-2351-1

THANET PRESS, MARGATE

Contents

1

Introduction

In writing this book I have attempted to follow the general pattern of the lectures which I have given to pupil midwives at Worcester Royal Infirmary for the past 21 years. In hospital it has been possible to illustrate what I have had to discuss by reference to cases at present in the wards. This unfortunately is not possible to the same extent in a book, but I have no doubt that my readers will be able to apply the principles described to cases under their care. I am sure that this is a most helpful way of fixing in one's mind the information which is required not only for examination purposes but so much more importantly for the better understanding of the clinical problems with which one is faced, and for the purpose of bringing to them the best possible management.

The chapter headings and the arrangement of the chapter content may be regarded as unorthodox, but I have presented the topics in the way in which they seem to me to arise in clinical practice. This, I hope, will make easier the understanding of all aspects of a problem. I have tried to avoid duplication, and when a topic appears in more than one place, it does so in order to discuss its relevance in a different context. Cross-references have been used throughout the text, in order to facilitate reference to the other facts of importance.

I hope that the guidance I have tried to give will prove helpful both to pupil midwives and to obstetric nurse students, and indirectly to their patients. This book is entitled 'Essential Obstetrics' and I have attempted to include all the information necessary for the practising midwife and to avoid the inclusion of irrelevant matter so that this may be a practical and concise textbook for members of the profession to which I have owed so much throughout my own professional lifetime.

It gives me pleasure to acknowledge the help which I have received from my son, Dr. I. G. de C. Chalmers, particularly in relation to the chapter entitled 'The foetus and his environment'.

2

The anatomy of reproduction

From the point of view of the obstetrician, the midwife and the obstetric nurse, the female pelvis is the bony channel through which the foetus has to make his way if he is to be delivered by the natural route, and it is the size and shape of the pelvis which imposes limitations upon the dimensions of the birth canal. A detailed understanding of the structure of the pelvis and its soft tissues is vital for the proper management of labour, and to help us distinguish the normal from the abnormal.

THE PELVIS

The pelvis consists of three compound bones, the sacrum which represents 5 modified vertebrae posteriorly and the two innominate bones on either side and extending round anteriorly. These three bones are joined together by the two sacro-iliac joints on either side posteriorly and the symphysis pubis in the mid-line anteriorly. All these three joints are normally virtually rigid in the non-pregnant woman, and this is of vital importance for the stability of the pelvis. During pregnancy, probably under the influence of a placental hormone called relaxin, all show an increased mobility which allows minor adaptation of the pelvis to the size and shape of the foetal head. The persistence of some of this mobility after pregnancy is over may lead to chronic low backache due to sacro-iliac subluxation.

The sacrum

The sacrum is roughly an inverted triangle, consisting of five fused sacral vertebrae (Fig.1). The lateral margins are formed by the fusion of the tips of the transverse processes, so as to leave four pairs of

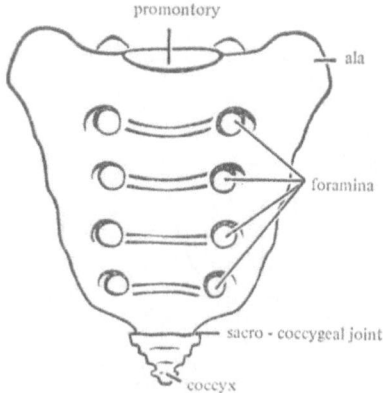

Fig.1. The sacrum.

sacral foramina, both anterior and posterior, through which the sacral vessels and nerves pass both forward into the pelvis and backwards into the lower back and gluteal regions. The bone is concave anteriorly, hollowed both from side to side and from above downwards; absence of this feature leads to diminution of the size of the pelvic cavity in certain contracted pelves.

The innominate or hip-bones

The innominate or hip-bones are irregular bones each comprising three elements which join together centrally to form the acetabulum, the strong cup-shaped depression which accommodates the head of the femur to form the hip joint (Fig.2). The uppermost bone is the *ilium*, a flattened blade concave antero-medially to form the iliac fossa, surmounted by a thickened ridge, the iliac crest. It tapers down to its heavy part which constitutes the upper two-fifths of the acetabulum. Below and posteriorly is the *ischium*, with a thickened tuberosity at its lower part which forms the lateral margin of the pelvic outlet. The bone extends up and forwards to form the lower two-fifths of the acetabulum, and medially the ischial spines jut to a variable extent towards the sacrum, at the level of the middle of the pelvic cavity. The third bone, the *pubis* has a more or less rectangular body on either side of the midline anteriorly, related to its fellow of the opposite side at the symphysis pubis. From its upper part, its superior ramus extends backwards to form the remaining anterior one-fifth of the acetabulum. From its lower margin, the

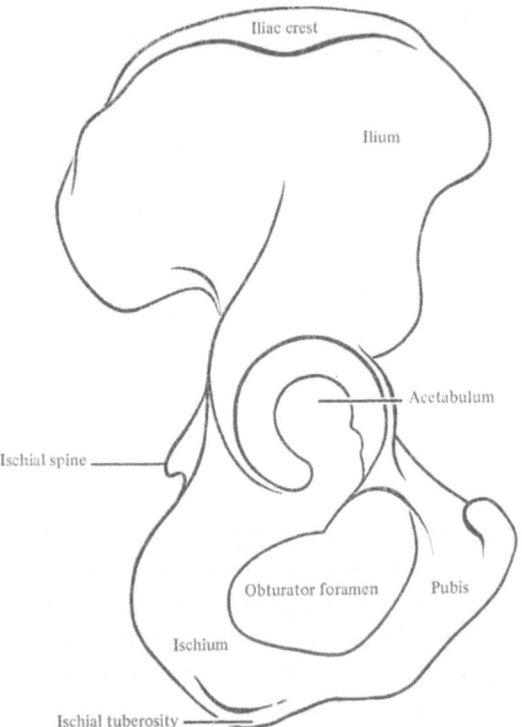

Fig.2. The innominate bone.

inferior ramus extends downwards and backwards towards the ischial tuberosity to form, with the inferior ramus of the opposite side, the pubic arch or sub-pubic angle.

The upper anterior margin of the body of the first sacral segment is described as the sacral promontory; above this the sacrum is related to the fifth lumbar vertebra. On either side of the promontory is the sacral ala or wing extending out to the sacro-iliac joint. At its lower end is the sacro-coccygeal joint where the sacrum articulates with the *coccyx*. The latter comprises the fused remnants of 3–5 coccygeal vertebrae, and these may move backwards and forwards at the hinged joint. This is sometimes ankylosed as the result of a heavy fall on the buttocks as for example at the edge of a swimming bath, but it rarely causes any obstruction to labour.

Pelvic diameters
A considerable number of pelvic diameters has been described, but

of these only a few are of real importance. The *pelvic brim or inlet* is a plane bounded by the sacral promontory behind and the ala of the sacrum on either side running round via the ileo-pectineal line to the upper margin of the symphysis pubis (Fig.3). The antero-

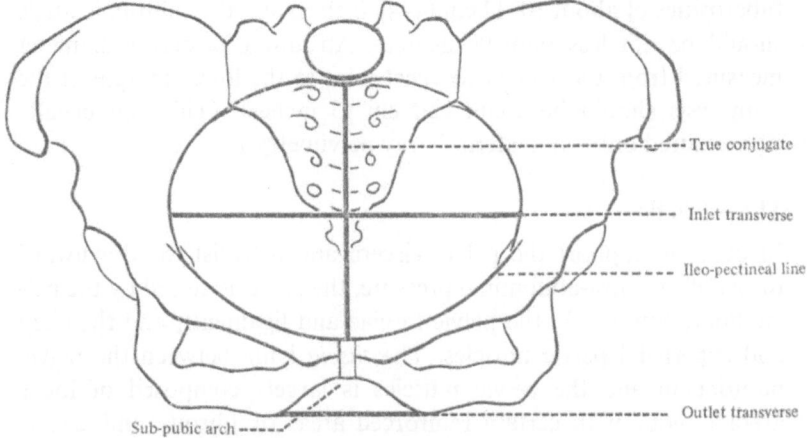

Fig.3. The pelvic brim.

posterior diameter of the brim, or true conjugate, extending from the sacral promontory to the upper margin of the symphysis, measures 10–11·5 cm (4–4½ inches) and the corresponding transverse diameter of the brim, the greatest distance between the lateral walls of the pelvis, is 12·5 cm (5 inches). Oblique diameters measured

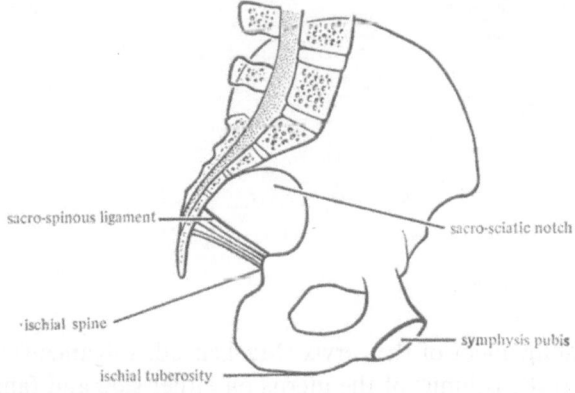

Fig.4. The pelvis—lateral view.

from their respective sacro-iliac joints usually amount to about 11·25 cm (4½ inches). The diameters of the *cavity* are less well-defined, but usually antero-posterior, transverse and oblique at this level are all about 11·25 cm (4½ inches). The *outlet*, the lower exit of the pelvis has a well-marked transverse diameter between the two ischial tuberosities of about 10–11 cm (4–4½ inches) and the sub-pubic angle should be not less than 90 degrees. An antero-posterior diameter measured from the sacro-coccygeal joint to the lower margin of the symphysis should be about 12·5 cm (5 inches). (This can usually be measured only on a lateral X-ray pelvimetry.)

The pelvic floor

In order to support the pelvic viscera and to resist the downward thrust of the intra-abdominal pressure, the pelvis is closed by the pelvic floor, comprising the pelvic fasciae and ligaments, and the deep and superficial pelvic muscles. The *fascia* lying between the pelvic peritoneum and the pelvic muscles is largely composed of loose areolar tissue with certain reinforced areas of fibrous and elastic tissue (Fig.5). The most important of these is the parametrium

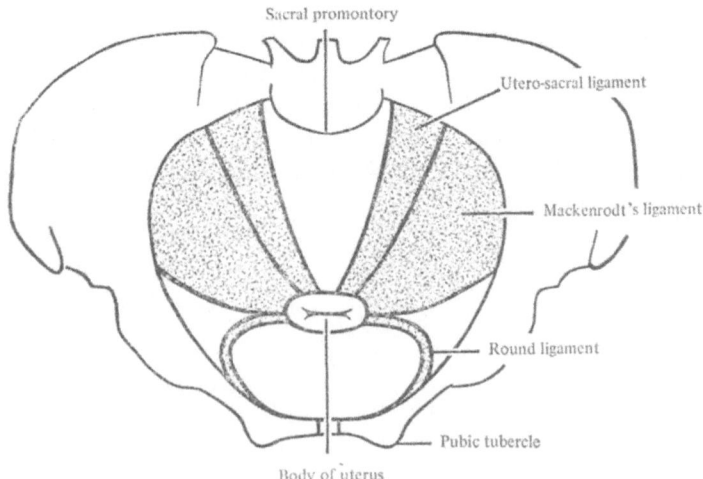

Fig.5. The pelvic fascia.

or cardinal ligament of the cervix (Mackenrodt's ligament) which is attached to the isthmus of the uterus on either side and fans out to be attached to the lateral pelvic wall. A posterior extension goes to the sacrum as the utero-sacral ligament and anteriorly, the utero-vesical ligament runs to the bladder. At a higher level, the round ligament runs from the uterine cornu laterally to the internal abdominal ring and then medially to be attached to the pubic tubercle near the upper margin of the symphysis. All of these ligaments help to suspend the uterus and its appendages and constitute a first line of defence in the prevention of prolapse, but they may be stretched by difficult or precipitate childbirth or by coughing or other increased intra-abdominal pressure. Should this occur, the second line defences are called into play, namely the *levatores ani*, comprising two sheets of muscle arising from the lateral pelvic wall and inserted into a median raphe through which pass the urethra and vagina in an anterior compartment and the anal canal posteriorly behind the perineal body (Fig.6). Contraction of these muscles elevates the median

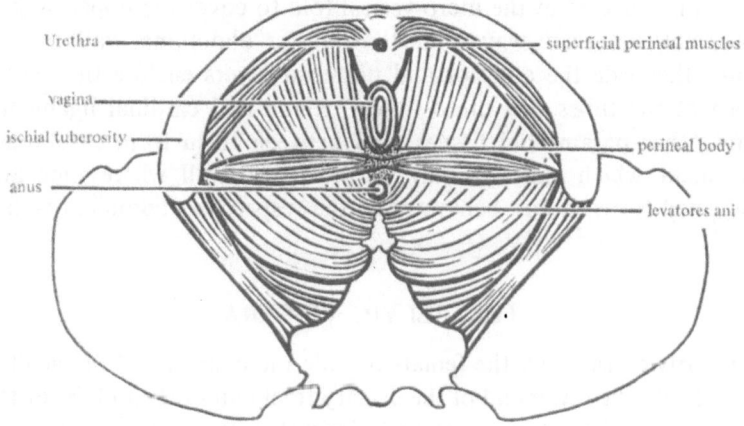

Fig.6. Muscles of the pelvic floor seen from below.

raphe and as their name implies, lifts up the anal canal so as to bring it into line with the lower rectum so as to facilitate defaecation, and at the same time, the muscles also prevent downward displacement of the pelvic viscera during straining. Below the level of the levators and between the lower vagina and the anal canal is the perineal body, a pyramidal mass of fibrous and elastic tissue which gives attachment to several of the *superficial perineal muscles*. Anteriorly these span the sub-pubic angle giving support to the lower vagina and the urethra, and include a vaginal sphincter, spasm of which (vaginismus) is a not infrequent cause of dyspareunia and has ruined

many a honeymoon. Posteriorly, the anal sphincter allows control of
bowel content—it may be damaged by extensive perineal tearing
during a precipitate or ill-managed delivery with disastrous results until it is accurately repaired. The interposition of the perineal body
between vagina and rectum fortunately prevents this mishap in all
but the most severe injuries.

The pelvic peritoneum

The pelvic peritoneum may be regarded as a sort of sheet dropped
down into the pelvis from above, hanging down both in front of and
behind the uterus and tubes as these stretch transversely across the
pelvis. Behind, the peritoneum extends right down over the back of
the uterus to form the pouch of Douglas before it is reflected upwards
over the anterior aspect of the rectum and the posterior abdominal
wall. In front, the uterine covering is only partial, since the peritoneum is reflected at the utero-vesical fold to cover the upper aspect
of the bladder on its way to line the anterior abdominal wall (Fig.8).
On either side the anterior and posterior layers enclose the major
part of the tubes, the utero-vesical, round and cardinal ligaments
and other parametrial tissues, and between them form the broad
ligament which runs laterally to the pelvic wall where they are
reflected forward and backward to the respective abdominal walls.

THE PELVIC VISCERA

The pelvic viscera in the female include the ovaries and the genital
tract, with the lower end of the urinary tract anteriorly and the distal
part of the alimentary canal posteriorly (Fig.7).

The ovary

The female gonad, the ovary, is usually described as almond-shaped
although there is much functional variation in both size and shape,
and is about 3 cm long, 2 cm broad and 1·5 cm thick. It is attached on
either side to the posterior leaf of the broad ligament, and its vessels
and nerves pass through from the pelvic connective tissue to reach
the ovarian hilum. At its medial end it is attached to the uterus by
the ovarian ligament; laterally it is suspended from the lateral pelvic
wall by the infundibulo-pelvic fold at the upper lateral margin of the
broad ligament. It is whitish or yellow in colour, usually with a
markedly convoluted surface cortex, the tunica albuginea.

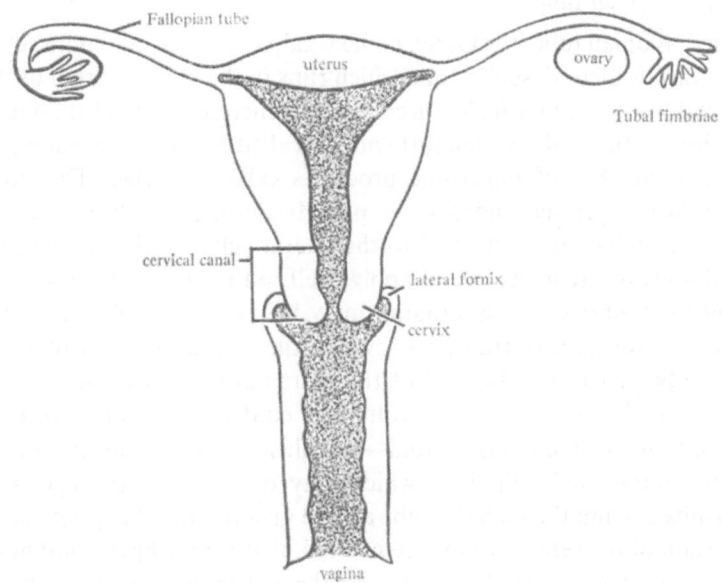

Fig.7. Internal genitalia in female.

The genital tract includes the Fallopian tubes on either side, the uterus and the vagina, which passes down through the pelvic floor beneath the pubic arch to emerge at the vulva. The genital tract is derived in the main from the Mullerian ducts, two tubes which lie side by side in the hind end of the body cavity of the early embryo, medial to a similar pair of tubes, the Wolffian ducts, which in the male are destined to form part of the sperm transport system of the genital tract. Should the chromosome pattern be female however (see below), the Wolffian ducts remain undeveloped and the Mullerian become dominant. The cephalad upper thirds form the Fallopian tube on each side, the middle thirds fuse together to form the uterus, whilst the lower thirds form the upper two-thirds of the vagina. The lower third of the vagina is formed by an invagination from below, the proctodaeum, which also gives rise to the anal canal. Failure of fusion may occur at any level, and this may give rise to various developmental abnormalities which are frequently encountered in obstetric departments such as bicornuate uterus, septate uterus, double uterus, etc., and which may be important in the obstetric management of the case.

The Fallopian tube

The Fallopian tube (the Greek name is salpinx, hence salpingitis, etc.) is a thin-walled muscular tube which runs in the upper margin of the broad ligament, by which it is completely enclosed except for an inch or less at the fimbrial (lateral) end, so called because it is equipped with a number of finger-like processes called fimbriae. The tube, like the ovary, is suspended at this point by the infundibulo-pelvic ligament by which it is attached to the lateral pelvic wall. The fimbrial end however, remains free to apply itself to the surface of the ovary, and the fimbriae in this situation may help to guide the ovum into the tube for onward transport towards the uterus. At its medial end the tube penetrates the wall of the uterus at its upper lateral part. The tube is lined with a tall columnar epithelium which is thrown up into many and complex folds—for this reason any infection may cause intra-tubal adhesions which may obstruct the passage of a fertilized ovum through the tube and so give rise to tubal pregnancy. Certain of the cells however are ciliated, that is they have small hair-like processes which beat towards the uterus and tend to sweep the ovum in this direction, an action which is further aided by tubal peristalsis also operating from fimbrial to uterine end.

The uterus

The uterus is a much more powerfully constructed organ than the tube, as might be expected when one considers the very different function which it may be called upon to perform. It is roughly pear-shaped, flattened from front to back, with its narrower portion downwards. Its overall length is about 7·5 cm (3 inches) and its upper end, the fundus, about 5·0 cm (2 inches) broad. Its thickness in the non-pregnant state is about 4·0 cm ($1\frac{1}{2}$ inches). The upper two thirds is called the body or corpus, the lower third the cervix. At each upper lateral angle is the uterine horn or cornu, where the tube enters and to which the round ligament is attached. The cavity of the non-pregnant uterus is triangular with anterior and posterior surfaces opposed and its lower apical portion communicates with the canal of the cervix, a thick-walled tube about 2·5 cm (one inch) long. At the upper end of this canal is the internal os and at the lower the external os or mouth of the cervix.

As we have seen above, the uterus is largely invested with peritoneum which posteriorly extends downwards as far as the upper (supra-vaginal) part of the cervix. Anteriorly however it passes forward to the bladder at about the level of the junction of body and cervix, the so-called isthmus uteri. Laterally the uterus is related to the tubes, to vessels and nerves between the layers of the broad ligament and to the cardinal and other ligaments described above.

The main bulk of the uterus is constituted by the myometrium, the muscle coat of the uterus, a plain muscle which has the property of reacting to oxytocic drugs, some of these hormonal in origin and others pharmacological. The arrangement of the myometrial muscle fibres is somewhat complex. In the body of the uterus many are longitudinal, to effect the expulsive function of this part of the organ, whilst other circular fibres play an adjuvant part in uterine peristalsis. Oblique fibres have also been described, as have highly specialized figure-of-eight fibres, whose particular function is to compress the large maternal blood vessels of the placental site and so to prevent haemorrhage after the separation of the placenta (see Chapter 12). In the cervix, on the other hand, the main musculature is circular, in accordance with the sphincteric action of the cervix, whose func-tion during pregnancy is largely to prevent expulsion of the uterine contents. There are also however longitudinal fibres, many extending down from the body, and contraction of these during labour tends to draw the cervix up over the presenting part so as to effect dilata-tion of the cervix. Throughout pregnancy, the corporeal myometrium should be at rest and the cervical circular fibres dominant; once labour begins, the cervix should relax and permit dilatation as a result of corporeal activity. This reciprocal relationship between body and cervix is described as polarity.

The uterine cavity is lined by a highly specialized epithelium called endometrium whose structure is modified during the different phases of the menstrual cycle, and which is largely shed at each menstrual flow and reformed thereafter (Chapter 3).

The uterus is normally angled forward upon itself (anteflexion) and also lies in such a position that the fundus points forwards and the cervix backwards and downwards (anteversion). The round ligaments above and in front, and the utero-sacral ligaments below and behind, help to maintain this position (Fig.8).

The cervix

The cervix projects backwards and downwards through the upper part of the anterior vaginal wall, that part which projects being called the vaginal portion of the cervix as distinct from the upper

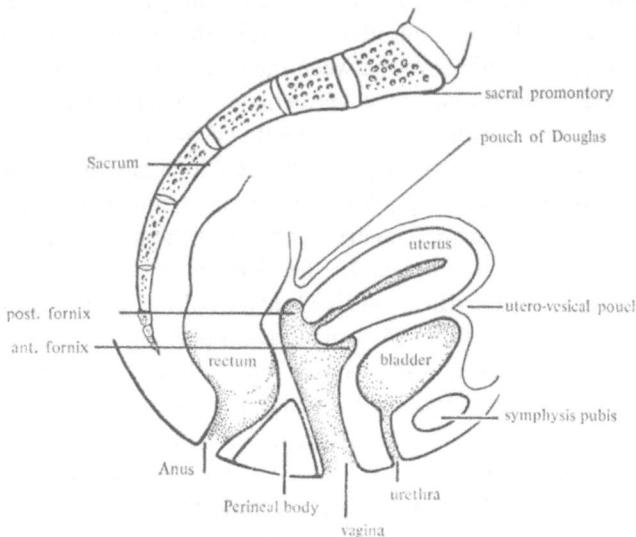

Fig.8. Pelvic viscera—lateral view.

supra-vaginal portion. Four recesses in front of and behind the cervix and on either side are described respectively as anterior, posterior and right and left lateral fornices. Through the posterior fornix one can palpate the contents of the pouch of Douglas and by means of the lateral fornices, the tube and ovary on either side (the adnexae or uterine appendages) may be palpated.

The vagina

The vagina is a fibro-muscular tube extending downwards and forwards from the cervix to the vulva. It is lined by a flattened squamous epithelium like that of the surface of the skin of the body, which is thrown up into folds which a romantically minded anatomist of the past called the arbor vitae or tree of life. It has a thin muscular coat and is capable of being very widely distended to permit the passage of the foetus. The anterior vaginal wall, about 7·5 cm (3 inches) long to the anterior fornix, is shorter than the posterior 11 cm (4½ inches) because the former is encroached upon by the cervix. It lies between the bladder and urethra in front and the rectum behind; the posterior fornix lies just below the peritoneal reflection at the pouch of Douglas. As we have seen, the perineal body is interposed between the lower vagina and the anal canal. The close relationship between the vagina and these other organs means that trauma to the vagina may easily extend to one of the others giving rise to fistula formation. Laterally the ischio-rectal fossa lies on either side, and although lateral vaginal trauma is not particularly common, haematomata or abscesses may sometimes occur in this situation after delivery.

The external female genitalia

The external female genitalia are described as the vulva, which lies in relation to the pubic angle at the lower end of the vagina (Fig.9).

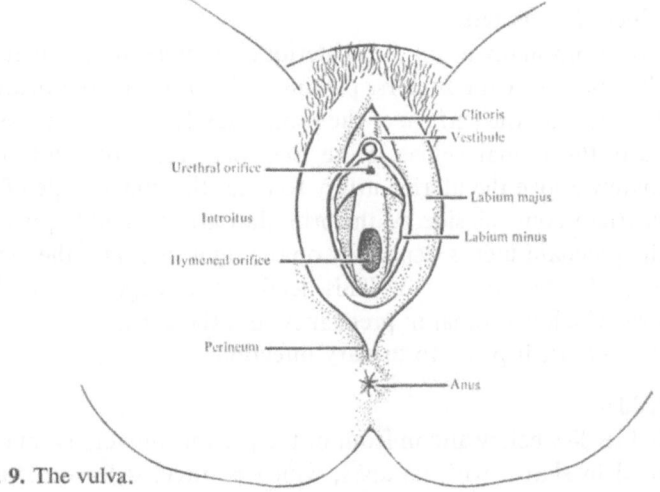

Fig. 9. The vulva.

It consists of two pairs of labia or lips, the larger, the labia majora, being rather fleshy masses lying on either side of the introitus, the entrance to the vagina. Anteriorly they fuse at the mons veneris, a fibro-fatty pad overlying the pubic bodies, and posteriorly they are joined by a skin fold, the posterior commissure or fourchette, which forms the anterior margin of the perineum. The labia minora are a pair of leaf-like structures which lie on the medial aspects of the labia minora. These pass anteriorly to a small triangular area in front of the introitus, known as the vestibule onto which opens the external urinary meatus. They then split to enclose the clitoris, the female homologue of the penis, a small erectile organ suspended below the symphysis by its suspensory ligament. The introitus in the virgin is partly occluded by the hymen, a membranous fold, commonly with a central orifice, which is usually torn at first coitus. The vulva is covered with skin and after puberty the lateral aspects of the labia majora and the mons veneris are covered with pubic hair.

The sigmoid colon

The sigmoid colon, by virtue of its mesocolon is so mobile that it may often lie in the pelvis and so be palpable on vaginal examination, often in the pouch of Douglas. The rectum lies in direct relation to the anterior surface of the sacrum, behind an anterior covering of peritoneum. Below the level of the pouch of Douglas and above the perineal body it is related to the middle third of the vagina. The anal canal lies at right angles to its lower end, turned backwards and downwards behind the perineal body.

The kidneys and ureters

The kidneys normally lie on the posterior abdominal wall well above the pelvic brim but the ureters, passing down towards the bladder, cross the brim on the surface of the psoas muscle to reach the pelvic floor near the ischial spines. Here they pass forwards and cross immediately above the uterine artery to enter the upper angle of the bladder trigone on each side. At the brim they are exposed to pressure from the pregnant uterus, especially on the right side since the uterus is commonly dextro-rotated. This leads to a degree of hydronephrosis which is normal in pregnancy, but the consequent stagnation of urine predisposes to urinary infection.

The bladder

The bladder lies below and in front of the peritoneum and is roughly pyramidal in shape, with its apex, which is directed forwards and slightly upwards, continuous with the urethra, which in the female is a narrow tube 4·5–5·0 cm ($1\frac{1}{2}$–2 inches) long passing below the pubic arch to open on the vestibule. The base of the bladder is in direct contact with the anterior vaginal wall and the supra-vaginal cervix and here lies the trigone, a smooth-walled, fixed triangular area, with the ureters entering at its upper angles and the urethra leaving the bladder at its lower angle. The remainder of the bladder is widely distensible and enlarged according to its content of urine. The urethro-vesical junction is suspended by the anterior fibres of the levator ani, and stretching of this muscle and the fascial ligaments above it may lead to prolapse and possibly to the very distressing symptom of stress incontinence.

The blood supply of the ovary

The blood supply of the ovary is derived from the ovarian artery, which runs down the posterior abdominal wall from the region of the kidney to reach the lateral pelvic wall, thence in the infundibulo-pelvic fold to the hilum of the ovary and on to anastomose with the ascending branch of the *uterine artery* in the region of the Fallopian tube which it also supplies. The uterine arteries are branches of the hypogastric division of the internal iliac artery and run across the pelvis above the ureter to the isthmus of the uterus, where they divide into ascending and descending branches. The former runs up the lateral border of the body of the uterus where it is very tortuous so as to permit rapid elongation when the uterus grows during pregnancy, and on below the tube to meet the ovarian artery. The descending branch supplies the cervix and upper part of the vagina. The vagina has a second supply via the vaginal branch of the internal iliac artery and a third from its internal pudendal branch. This vessel also supplies the vulva along with the external pudendal branch of the femoral artery. The venous drainage corresponds broadly with the arterial supply. It is noteworthy however that a large plexus of veins lies in the posterior end of the labium majus on each side; this becomes greatly distended during pregnancy and then may not only give rise to aching and uncomfortable varicose veins, but may also be the source of a large vulval haematoma as a result of quite minor trauma during delivery.

THE FOETAL SKULL

For the obstetrician and the midwife, the foetal skull is the largest part of the foetus at term; that is to say, if the foetal skull can pass through the birth canal the remainder of the body should follow

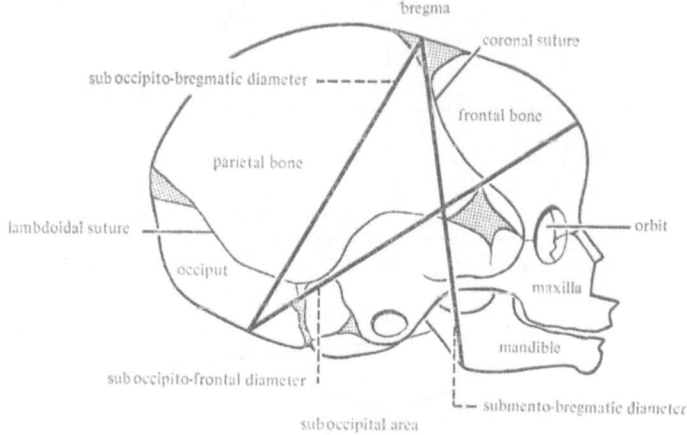

Fig.10. The foetal skull.

without difficulty. This is true of all foetuses of average size; in very
large foetuses however, the bisacromial diameter across the shoulders
may be wider than any of the skull diameters and may give rise to
difficulty in delivery of the shoulders—so-called shoulder dystocia,
which can present such a problem in a foetus over about 4·100G
(9·0 lbs) in weight (Fig.10).

The skull may be regarded as comprising the face and base, both
composed of rather massive, firmly united and incompressible bones,
and the cranium or vault, which consists of five bones which are
not only thin and compressible but are united only by membranous
sutures. As a result, the shape of the head may be altered by compression during its passage through the birth canal, bones tending
to overlap the adjacent bones at their sutures (moulding). This may
lead to reduction in one diameter but at the same time there is a
compensatory increase in another, and the total skull volume is not
decreased. Excessive moulding is usually an indication of disproportion and may be associated with tearing of intra-cranial membranes with consequent haemorrhage.

The vault

We need not consider the base of the skull or the face in detail, but
further study of the vault will be helpful (Fig.11). The vault consists
of five bones, two pairs and an unpaired bone. Anteriorly lie the

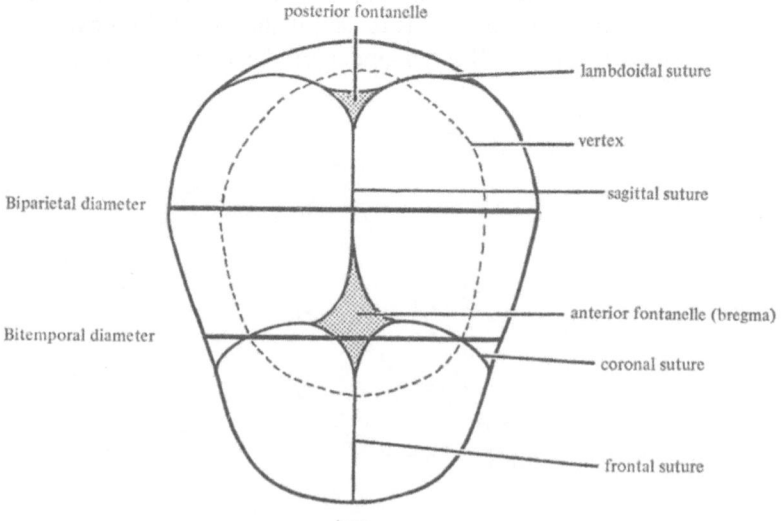

Fig.11. The vault of the skull.

frontal bones joined in the middle line by the frontal suture. On either side of the vault lies the parietal bone, united to the frontal bones by the coronal suture, and to the opposite parietal by the sagittal suture. Posteriorly lies the single occipital bone, united to the two parietal bones by the L-shaped lambdoidal suture. At the junction of the frontal, sagittal and coronal sutures is a diamond-shaped area of membrane described as the anterior fontanelle or bregma, and posteriorly, where the sagittal suture meets the angle of the lambdoidal, is the posterior fontanelle which is usually much smaller than the anterior. It is usually easy to distinguish the triradiate form of the posterior from the four-cornered anterior fontanelle, and on vaginal examination in labour it is usually easily palpable if the well-flexed head is presenting. If one can reach the anterior fontanelle this indicates deflexion of the head such as occurs in occipito-posterior positions. The area between the two fontanelles and on either side of the sagittal suture is described as the vertex.

All these cranial bones are similar in shape, with an external convexity rising to an apex variously described as the frontal eminence, the parietal eminence and the occipital protruberance. The area below the last named is the suboccipital area and two important skull diameters are measured from this point.

Skull diameters
The most important transverse diameter of the skull, because it is the widest, is the biparietal, the distance between the two parietal eminences, normally 9·5 cm (3·75 inches). The bitemporal diameter of 8·0 cm (3·25 inches) lies between the furthest points of the coronal suture.

The most important antero-posterior diameters of the skull, because they are the smallest, are the suboccipito-bregmatic and the submento-bregmatic, each measuring 9·5 cm (3·75 inches), and which, together with the biparietal diameter, are the presenting diameters with a well-flexed vertex and a face presentation respectively. The suboccipito-frontal diameter of 10 cm (4 inches) presents with a somewhat deflexed occipito-posterior vertex. The mento-vertical of 13·5 cm (5·5 inches) is longer than any diameter of the pelvic brim; it presents in a brow presentation and if foetus and pelvis are of average size, normal birth is impossible.

THE BREASTS
The breasts in the female are a pair of glandular swellings on the front of the chest wall lying over the pectoral muscles, principally

pectoralis major, between the 2nd and the 6th ribs, and extending from the lateral border of the sternum of the mid-axillary line. An extension from the upper lateral quadrant up into the axilla is described as the axillary tail. In the centre of each breast is a circular area of pigmented skin about 2·5 cm (1 inch) in diameter, called the *areola*, and in the centre of this again a raised mass of erectile tissue about 0·5 cm ($\frac{1}{4}$ inch) in diameter called the *nipple*. On the surface of the nipple are the openings of 18–20 *lactiferous ducts*. Each duct drains the secretion of the *alveoli*, the functioning glands of the breast. The alveoli of each of the 18–20 lobes of the breast secrete colostrum during pregnancy into a small reservoir deep to the nipple called the ampulla. Here it is stored until the breast secretion is expressed, or suckling takes place, when it reaches the exterior via the ducts. Apart from these glandular tissues and ducts the breasts contain a variable amount of fat (Fig.12). Changes occurring in the breast during pregnancy are discussed in Chapter 4 and those during the puerperium in Chapter 7.

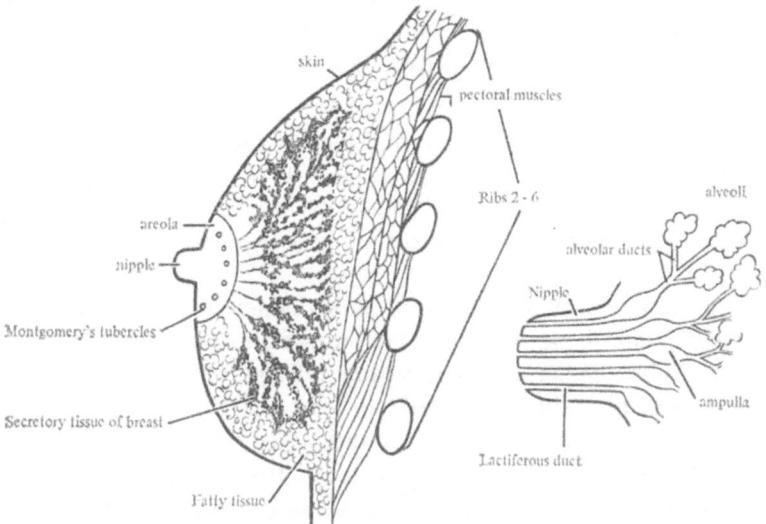

Fig.12. The breast.

3

The physiology of reproduction

THE OVARIAN CYCLE

During the early years of life, although in the normal individual the basis of sexual development is already laid down, the various genital organs described in the preceding chapter are in an immature, resting stage. At puberty, however, various hormonal changes occur which begin the process of bringing these organs and indeed the whole body to a state of full functional maturity. It is the ovarian hormone oestrogen which in the female at about the age of 10–14 years effects the development of the secondary sex characters and growth and maturation of the genital organs. The development of the breasts, the acquisition of the feminine figure, the appearance of pubic and axillary hair and the growth in size and vascularity of both internal and external genital organs all occur as a result of the secretion of this hormone.

It is not yet clear what is the trigger mechanism which sets in train the sequence of events which leads to these changes and to the eventual occurrence of menstruation, but it is known that the hypothalamus secretes two separate releasing hormones, at present called follicle stimulating hormone releasing hormone (FSHRH) and luteinising hormone releasing hormone (LHRH). These act upon the anterior lobe of the pituitary gland to effect release of the pituitary gonadotrophins, follicle stimulating hormone (FSH) and luteinising hormone (LH). The former, FSH, in turn leads to development in the ovary of the Graafian follicle which secretes oestrogen and eventually ruptures to release the ovum (ovulation), whilst the latter, LH, causes transformation of the follicle at this stage to the corpus luteum, which secretes not only oestrogen but also progesterone (Fig.15).

Ovulation

The ovary contains within its rather tough cortex a prodigious number of tiny structures called primordial follicles, each in theory capable of production of an ovum and ultimately of a pregnancy. Happily, the enormous majority of these never develop, else the population explosion would be a veritable cataclysm! Each month, however, one follicle is selected for development (it is not known how this selection occurs) and under the influence of FSH it grows to become a cystic structure of about 1–1·5 cm in diameter lined with an outer layer of theca cells and two or more layers of granulosa cells, and containing clear fluid. At one point on its internal surface is a small mass, the cumulus oophorus, where the granulosa cells are heaped up around the developing ovum. The follicle, now described as the *Graafian follicle* (Fig.13), migrates to the surface of the ovary

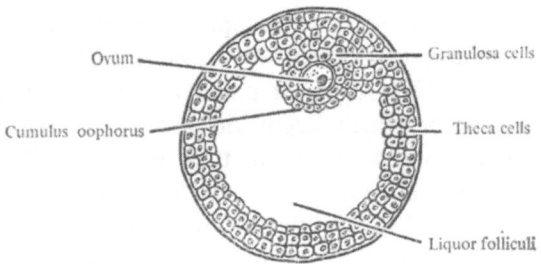

Ovum — Granulosa cells
Cumulus oophorus — Theca cells
Liquor folliculi

Fig.13. The Graafian follicle.

where it ruptures, releasing the ovum surrounded by some of its granulosa cells, into the peritoneal cavity. Here, if circumstances are favourable, the fimbrial end of the Fallopian tube is awaiting it, applied to the appropriate point on the surface of the ovary. The ovum is guided into the lumen of the tube and is carried both by peristalsis and by ciliary action towards the uterus.

In the ovary, the follicle now seals itself off, and under the influence of LH is converted into a *corpus luteum* (yellow body), a slightly larger structure (2·0–2·5 cm) lined with the large yellow cells from which it takes its name (Fig.14). This secretes not only oestrogen but also the second of the ovarian hormones, progesterone. Unlike the Graafian follicle, its lining is thickened and convoluted and the central cavity often contains some blood.

At this point, the oestrogen and progesterone levels in the blood

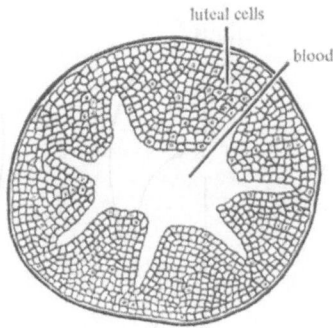

Fig.14. The corpus luteum.

are raised to such an extent that, through an inhibitory feed-back mechanism, the anterior pituitary hormones, FSH and LH are no longer produced (Fig.15). Hence stimulation of the ovary is cut off until regression of the corpus luteum occurs, with a resultant fall in oestrogen and progesterone levels. This permits renewed secretion of FSH and LH, ovarian stimulation is resumed and a new Graafian follicle is developed.

Changes in the uterus

Meanwhile, in the uterus, striking changes are occurring. The secretion of oestrogen by the ovary is followed by development of the vascular supply of the uterus which leads to growth of the whole organ. The myometrium becomes much thicker and develops its adult pattern. The most remarkable changes however affect the endometrium. Before puberty, this epithelium lining the cavity of the uterus is thin, poorly vascularized and with only a few tiny glands. Once oestrogen is available however the endometrium becomes much thicker, with improved blood supply and a great increase in the number and size of the glands, which however in this, the *proliferative phase*, are comparatively simple in form and devoid of secretion. After ovulation, with the availability of progesterone as well as oestrogen, the endometrium becomes still more vascular, the glands larger and now serrated in shape, with droplets of secretion visible in the cells lining them, giving this the name, the *secretory phase*. The differences between these two endometrial phases are usually so clear-cut that it is possible to establish by examination of endometrial curettings whether or not ovulation has

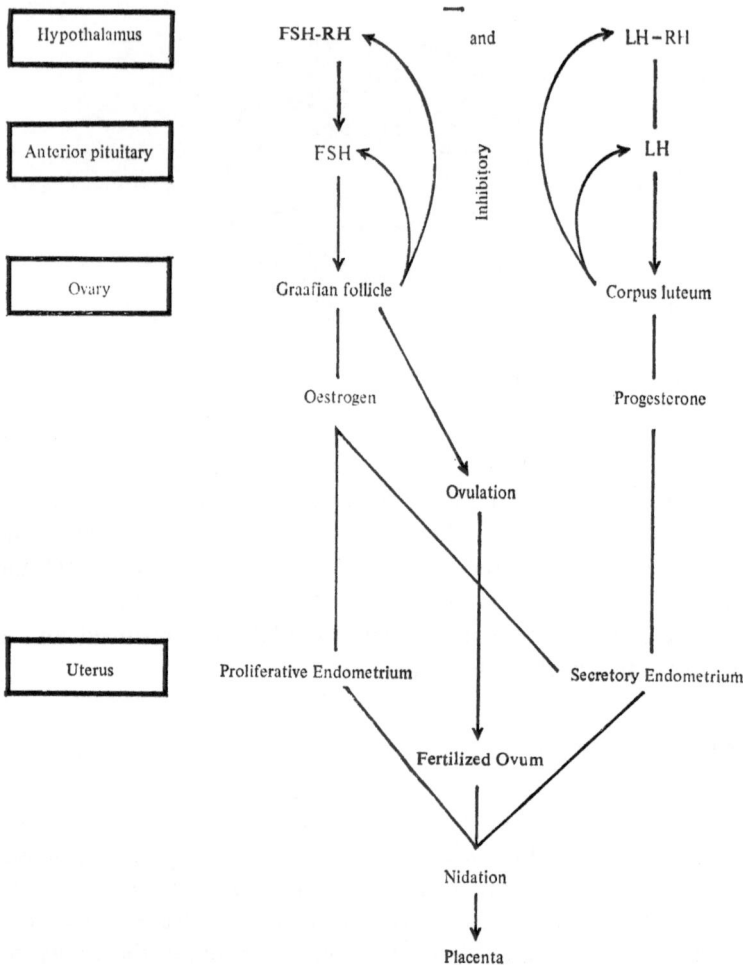

Fig.15. The endocrine control of establishment of pregnancy.

occurred, and this is of course of great value in the investigation of infertility.

The cervical canal is lined with highly complex branching glands which secrete mucus. This mucus is thick and tenacious but under the influence of oestrogen becomes clear and watery at the time of ovulation, so as to allow the sperms access to the upper genital tract when on their way to fertilize the ovum. At other times the mucus plug effectively blocks the cervical canal and helps to prevent ascending infection. Occasionally however infection may lurk in the depths of some of the branching glands, and this may be important if the infecting organism is the gonococcus which may reach the eyes of the foetus during delivery and cause a disastrous ophthalmia (Chapter 18).

The menstrual cycle

In the light of all the foregoing it is now possible to consider the significance of the menstrual cycle, which occurs from the onset of menstruation (menarche) to the menopause. In the early years after puberty and in the last few years before the menopause, menstruation may be anovulatory, i.e. neither ovulation, corpus luteum formation nor progesterone secretion will occur. This is one reason why pregnancy is comparatively rare in these age groups and why heavy and prolonged bleeding is often found. For most of the period of active sexual life, however, the full endocrine cycle with ovulation and all the consequential changes occur about once a month, in most women, with a cycle of about 28 days. The menstrual cycle may be regarded as a preparation for pregnancy—if pregnancy does not occur all the changes brought about will regress only to be repeated in the next cycle. The menstrual period is a sort of cleaning-up process. Following the inhibition of secretion of anterior pituitary hormones, the corpus luteum will regress, and levels of oestrogen and progesterone will fall away. This in turn will lead to necrosis of the endometrium, which will be shed together with a variable amount of blood over several days. After the superficial five-sixths or thereabouts of the endometrium has been shed, only a thin basal layer of relatively inactive tissue is left attached to the myometrium. By this time however the new Graafian follicle is already secreting oestrogen, the FSH secretion having been re-established by the fall in oestrogen levels, and so the repair and proliferative development of the endometrium begin within a day or two of onset of the cycle. The first day of loss is described as day one, and the proliferative phase lasts until day 14. At this stage ovulation occurs and the corpus luteum is formed. This lasts about 10–12 days, when it regresses as we have seen; necrosis of the endometrium follows in about 48 hours, and so the next menstrual flow ensues after a total of 28 days. Where the menstrual cycle is longer or shorter than 28 days, there is little or no variation in length of the luteal phase of the cycle, i.e. ovulation almost always occurs about 14 days before the next period, and if conception occurs it generally does so within 24 hours of this point. With a 21 day cycle therefore, one would expect ovulation and conception about day 7, with a 35 days cycle about day 21, necessitating a corresponding modification of calculations regarding the duration of pregnancy.

Each menstrual period may be considered to result from failure to conceive and so we may now proceed to consider what happens when conception occurs.

Conception

Each animal species derives its hereditary characteristics from both parents by means of portions of nuclear chromatin called chromosomes. Each chromosome carries large numbers of genes which determine to what extent the offspring will resemble one or other parent. Some genes are dominant and others recessive, and of corresponding genes derived from each parent, the dominant will produce the appropriate characteristic in the offspring. A recessive gene however, if paired with another recessive gene may be expressed as a characteristic of the offspring. The child may therefore have his father's hair, his mother's eyes, etc., according to the dominance of the relevant genes.

Each species has its own characteristic number of chromosomes, the human figure being 46. These are comprised of 22 pairs plus two sex chromosomes. The paired chromosomes have been derived equally from the two parents to carry the relevant genes as we have seen above. The sex chromosomes are described as X and Y; if both sex chromosomes are X, the individual carrying them will be female, if one is X and the other Y, he will be male. The mother being female with an XX pattern can only pass on an X chromosome to her child; the father being XY, may pass either X or Y, and so it is he who determines the sex of the child.

The chromosome pattern of any individual is described as the karyotype, and in the normal human female this may be described as 46 XX; in the male it will be 46 XY—if there is any variation from this, the individual will be abnormally developed, usually sterile and often incapable of survival—for example the 47 XX type, who has 3 instead of 2 chromosomes of pair 21, will be a female mongol suffering from Down's syndrome.

The nucleus of each cell of the body in the normal individual will carry 46 chromosomes. When conception occurs, the ovum and the sperm must each contribute 23. This is effected during the maturation of both ovum and sperm. When a somatic cell divides, it does so by *mitosis*, i.e. each chromosome splits into two, so that each daughter cell will have 46 chromosomes just as does the parent cell. When the ovum is shed from the follicle, it has 46 chromosomes, but now it undergoes *meiosis*, or reduction division, to produce a mature ovum with 23 chromosomes, one of each pair and one X sex chromosome going to each daughter cell. Of these daughter cells, one will be a polar body, which is absorbed and has no further importance whilst the other, the mature ovum, is ripe for fertilization.

The spermatozoon is the corresponding male element, and is eventually formed as the result of a series of transformations of cells from the testes, respectively the spermatogonium, the primary spermatocyte and the secondary spermatocyte. This last undergoes reduction division so that the spermatozoon contains 23 chromosomes, one from each pair plus either an X or a Y sex chromosome.

The provision of spermatozoa is even more prodigal than that of potential ova, and each seminal ejaculate contains many millions of these cells. At intercourse semen is deposited in the posterior vaginal fornix and if conditions are favourable, i.e. if the cervical mucus is clear and fluid, indicating recent or impending ovulation, very large numbers of sperms will enter the cervical canal, and will make their way up the genital tract and into the tube, moving anti-dromically against the tide both of ciliary activity and of tubal peristalsis. Of all these cells, one only will reach the ovum and penetrate its cell membrane so that their nuclei will fuse and the characteristic number of 46 chromosomes be restored. According to whether the fertilizing sperm bears an X or a Y chromosome, the resultant offspring will be female or male (Fig.16). The remaining sperms will die and be discharged from the genital tract.

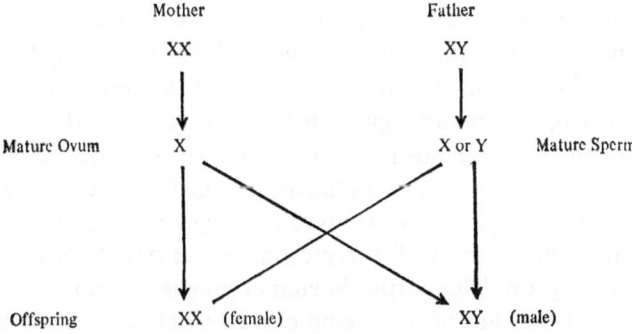

Fig.16. Chromosomal determination of sex.

Development of the fertilized ovum

Fertilization usually occurs in the wide ampullary portion of the tube towards its fimbrial end, and the fertilized ovum now continues on its way to the uterus, which it should reach about 6–7 days after ovulation. By this time, the corpus luteum should be well-formed and the progesterone-influenced endometrium in a well-developed secretory phase, so that it is capable of both embedding and nourishing the fertilized ovum. The ovum invades the superficial part of the endometrium, usually on either the anterior or posterior surface of the cavity of the uterus; the endometrium soon grows over the point of entry to cover it over. By this time, many changes have taken place in the ovum itself as a result of cell division. First the single-celled ovum divides into 2, 4, 8 etc. identical daughter cells eventually to form a bunch of similar cells called the morula from its resemblance to the mulberry fruit. This later becomes cystic with a fluid-filled central cavity, and it is now described as a blastocyst. From this stage cell specialisation is clearly recognized. On the surface of the blastocyst is the primitive trophoblast from which the chorion will later develop. At first the whole surface of the blastocyst is covered with spines like those on a horse-chestnut, each of them consisting of a chorionic villus, a hair-like process with a cellular inner covering, the Langhans layer, and superficially a curious structure called the syncytium or syncytio-trophoblast, a web of protoplasm with many nuclei scattered about. This has the property of invasiveness and helps the ovum to embed itself in the endometrium. Some of the chorionic villi, the nutrient villi, have central vessels, and when these invade maternal sinuses in the uterine wall they enable exchange of gases, foodstuffs, antibodies, products of metabolism etc. between maternal and foetal blood-streams which are separated only by the trophoblastic cells. Other villi have no vessels and have an anchoring function only, enabling the ovum to fix itself to the uterine wall. As the pregnancy advances the villi over much of the surface of the ovum atrophy, whilst those over about one-sixth of the surface proliferate and hypertrophy, and are aggregated together to form the placenta.

Although the mechanism is not yet clearly understood, once a fertilized ovum is established in the uterus, the feed-back mechanism inhibiting the secretion of FSH and LH is suppressed, and as a result the corpus luteum, instead of regressing about day 26 of the cycle, continues to grow. This corpus luteum of pregnancy, as it is called to distinguish from the corpus luteum of menstruation, is much larger, up to 5 cm diameter, and secretes greatly increased amounts of oestrogen and progesterone until about the twelfth week, when this function is taken over by the placenta which should be well-developed by this time. As a result of the increased blood levels of the ovarian hormones, the endometrium is developed beyond its secretory phase to form the decidua, which is thicker, more vascular and more richly supplied with glands with markedly oedematous stromal cells (decidual cells). This tissue is responsible for the further development and support of the ovum at this stage and various elements of decidua are described. That part of the decidua lying between the ovum and the myometrium is the decidua basalis, whilst that separating the ovum from the uterine cavity is called the decidua capsularis. The remainder of the decidua lining the uterine cavity is the decidua vera. As the ovum grows, both D. basalis and D. capsularis increase at the expense of D. vera, until about the twelfth week of pregnancy, the D. capsularis fuses with the D. vera as the ovum fills the uterine cavity.

Within the ovum itself, some weeks before these changes have occurred, certain important changes have been taking place. A cavity, the amniotic sac, appears in the wall of the blastocyst as a thickened point called the embryonic area and displaces the embryonic plate towards the centre of the blastocyst (Fig.17). This plate is

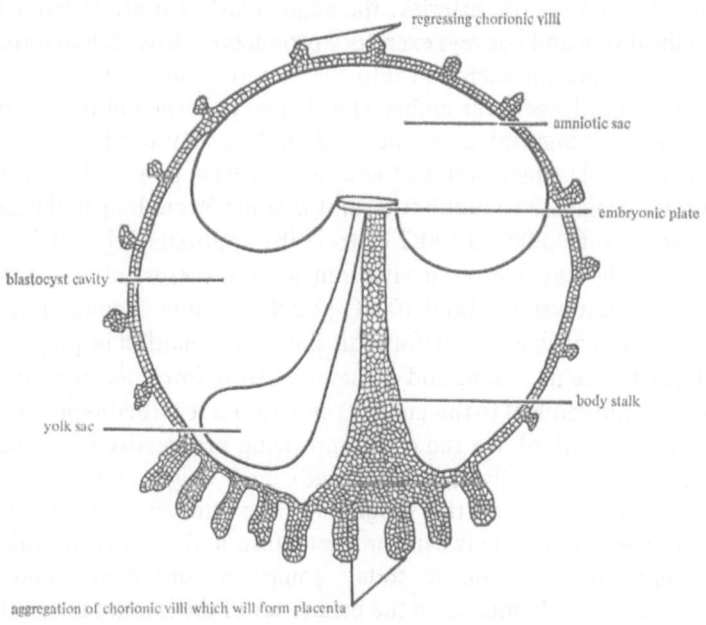

Fig.17. The developing ovum about the twelfth day.

2

comprised of three layers of cells, the ectoderm, which gives rise to all superficial structures of the body, the skin, hair and nails as well as the central nervous system, the mesoderm from which develop the bones, muscles, heart and blood vessels, kidneys, urinary tract, internal genital organs including the gonads and endocrine glands, and the entoderm from which the alimentary tract and many of its glands such as the liver are derived. The amniotic cavity is lined by the amnion which secretes the liquor amnii and as this increases in size it encircles the embryonic plate which then comes to lie within the cavity remaining attached to the chorion by the body-stalk which later becomes the umbilical cord. Alongside this is another meso-dermal structure the yolk-sac which contains albuminoid material and communicates directly with the primitive gut for which it acts as a reservoir of nutrient material. As this is gradually consumed the yolk-sac dwindles, so the amniotic sac increases to occupy the whole of the blastocyst cavity; the remnant of the yolk-sac persists only as a thin tube in the structure of the body stalk.

Once the placenta has developed, the vessels of the chorionic villi fuse together to form large trunks coursing over the foetal surface of the placenta, where they join to form the two arteries of the umbili-cal cord. These carry oxygen and nutrients to the foetus where they enter the hypogastric arteries; the single cord vein arises from the umbilical vein and conveys excretory products such as carbon dioxide to the placenta for excretion into the maternal blood-stream.

By the third week, the embryo has begun to form and by the sixth a foetus is recognizable and about 2 cm long. By the twelfth week limbs are well formed and the foetus is some 9 cm long, and thereafter it grows progressively until at term it is some 50 cm long and weighs on the average 3,000–3,500G (7 to 7½ lbs approximately). It is said to be viable (capable of survival outside the uterus) after the 28th week, when it weighs about 1000G (2·2 lbs), although comparatively few such infants survive. Before this point, termination of pregnancy is regarded as abortion, and a foetus born before this stage rarely survives. Subsequent to this stage termination is regarded as premature labour, the outlook for the child improving progressively as term is approached, especially once the infant's birth weight exceeds 2,500G (5½ lbs). For a long time this weight has been internationally accepted as the dividing line between the premature and the mature infant, although this criterion is today somewhat discredited and an assessment based more upon the behaviour of the infant preferred.

4

Diagnosis of pregnancy

INITIAL INDICATIONS OF PREGNANCY

1. *Failure to menstruate.* The first sign that draws a woman's attention to the fact that she may be pregnant is the failure of an expected menstrual period to appear. This is by no means diagnostic, but where menstruation has previously been regular it is probably significant. In many women however menstruation is irregular with occasional missed periods, and there are many causes of amenorrhoea other than pregnancy such as pituitary tumours, the Stein-Leventhal syndrome, functioning ovarian tumours, etc. Again amenorrhoea is normal before puberty and after the menopause and even this may sometimes give rise to confusion.

2. *Breast changes.* In the early stages, breast changes are often helpful. The breasts develop rapidly under the influence of the increased oestrogen secretion, and from about twelve weeks secretion of colostrum, a clear fluid containing lactose in solution, may occur and this may be expressed from the breasts. Earlier than this, from about 7–8 weeks after the first day of the last menstrual period (LMP), they may become tense and painful, and the mother may complain of tingling and tenderness. Inspection will show an increase in vascularity with bluish veins coursing across the surface of the breasts (marbling). The nipple and its areola will be pigmented, the degree of pigmentation corresponding to the general colouring of the woman. Around the areola about 16–24 small papillae may be observed; these are Montgomery's tubercles (Fig.12) and represent sebaceous glands whose function is to lubricate the skin of the areola and toughen it in preparation for lactation.

3. *Pregnancy sickness*. Soon after the first period is missed, pregnancy sickness may appear. Typically this may occur on waking in the morning but in some women may be troublesome in the evening and in the less fortunate may persist throughout the day and even the night (see Chapter 5). Whilst this symptom is present in about 75 per cent of women to a greater or less extent, it may be completely absent in the remainder.

4. *Frequency of micturition* is often complained of in the second month, owing probably to slight displacement of the bladder neck area as the uterus begins to grow. Late in pregnancy, frequency and even stress incontinence may again be troublesome as the presenting part presses upon the bladder as it enters the pelvic brim.

5. *Psychological changes* include emotional instability and vasomotor instability may lead to fainting and giddiness. Strange cravings for rather bizarre articles of diet have been reported, and some women recognize that they are pregnant because they can no longer tolerate alcohol or tobacco.

6. *Changes in the uterus, vagina and cervix.* Examination of the patient in the early weeks will show the breast changes described from about 7 weeks. A uterine mass arising out of the pelvis may be palpable in some thin and well-relaxed women as early as 8 weeks, but in their more generously-proportioned sisters it may be impossible to feel the uterus until the twelfth week, when it should be rising to 3 finger breadths above the symphysis pubis. Even this may be confused by the presence of fibroids or other pelvic tumours.

On vaginal examination, a bluish colouration of both the vaginal walls and the cervix may be observed from about the sixth week and soon after this, softening of the cervix which has the consistency of the lip rather than the nose in contrast to the non-pregnant cervix. The uterus can be felt to be enlarged and cystic from about the sixth week, but this finding may be doubtful in the obese patient before the tenth week.

7. *Changes in the urine.* Pregnancy testing of the urine is widely used today and is based upon the greatly increased excretion of gonadotrophins in the urine. These are largely secreted by the developing placenta and this continues increasingly until the placental activity falls off towards the end of pregnancy. The animal tests using

mice, rats, rabbits, frogs, toads, etc, have been almost completely replaced by immunological tests using latex particles or sheep's red cells sensitized to the hormones. These tests are highly reliable; in cases where the output of gonadotrophins is low, false negatives may be obtained, but false positive results are very rare. The tests are of little value before about the sixth week, and are best carried out on the first morning specimen which tends to have the highest concentration of hormones. The tests may be used not only for the diagnosis of pregnancy but also to determine whether in a disturbed pregnancy the foetus is still alive with a functioning placenta, and quantitative tests are helpful in the diagnosis of hydatidiform mole.

In most cases, clinical diagnosis of pregnancy should be possible with certainty by about the twelfth week, although a strong presumptive diagnosis should often be possible much earlier if a summation of all the available evidence is made.

ADVANCED PREGNANCY

As the pregnancy advances, further indications will become available. The continued growth of the abdominal mass to correspond with the dates may be observed, and the height of the fundus uteri to be expected at different key stages is indicated in Figure 18. It must however be realized that not only does the level of the umbilicus vary in different women, but that in some the uterus lies relatively high and in others lower. Where the fundal height does not correspond to the dates, therefore, careful palpation of the uterine mass may give a better idea of the duration of pregnancy than the fundal height alone.

At about the twentieth week of pregnancy in a woman pregnant for the first time (primigravida) and at 18 weeks or earlier in a woman who has previously borne a child (multipara), foetal movements should be felt (quickening). Some women will deny movements even when they are clearly palpable to the observer, and of course absence of movements may indicate foetal death. In general however, the date of quickening is a remarkably good guide to the stage which the pregnancy has reached.

The foetal heart may become audible between 24 and 28 weeks with the ordinary foetal stethoscope and some observers may be able to hear it even earlier. With electronic instruments such as the

Sonic Aid or Doptone foetal blood flow detectors, it may be recognized as early as the twelfth week. It may be inaudible as a result of gross obesity, of intra-uterine death or because of the absence of pregnancy.

Foetal parts can usually be palpated by 24 weeks, and in particular the small head may often be felt at the fundus, since breech presentation occurs at this stage of pregnancy. Ballottement may be elicited, that is the head may be felt to float back against the fingers if it has been gently tapped away.

As the pregnancy advances still further, there should be little difficulty in recognizing the foetal parts and in hearing the foetal heart, but even now, in the last weeks of pregnancy, doubt may remain especially if the patient is particularly obese or if the abdominal mass does not correspond with the dates.

In such a case, radiological investigation may be justified although it does carry certain risks for the foetus such as the later development of juvenile leukaemia. X-radiation is particularly harmful during the period of organogenesis, that is when the various organs, especially the sense organs, are in process of formation, around the sixth to the fourteenth week. If radiology is required it is probably best restricted to the third trimester (three-month period) and the dose of radiation kept as low as possible. Hence, although foetal bones may be recognized as early as the fourteenth week, it is rarely justifiable to use this method of investigation before about the twenty-ninth week.

Occasionally the diagnosis of pregnancy is not made until the patient is actually in labour and in such cases it may be difficult to persuade her that she is pregnant until the delivery of her baby is demonstrated to her. On the other hand, in pseudocyesis (false pregnancy), as a result of either wishful thinking or of guilty apprehension, the patient may wrongly believe herself to be pregnant. In such cases, the abdomen may be greatly distended but the size does not usually correspond to dates and breast and other signs are absent. The diagnosis is not usually difficult but should not be lightly made, as it may greatly distress the patient. On the other hand the earlier it is made, the less distress is likely to persist.

5

Ante-natal care

THE PURPOSE OF ANTE-NATAL CARE

The purposes of ante-natal care are to observe the general health and condition of the pregnant woman, to detect at an early stage any deviations from the normal, to make whatsoever provision is necessary to bring the patient to the end of her pregnancy in the best possible condition and to ensure that the place of her delivery offers the greatest safety for mother and baby. Little ante-natal care was undertaken before the beginning of the present century, but since then and particularly since 1945, there has been such a great increase in facilities that few women do not receive more or less adequate supervison during pregnancy.

There is at present a strong movement towards 100 per cent hospital confinement and domiciliary delivery is becoming less and less frequent. The many general practitioner maternity units can make a valuable contribution towards the care of the normal case, but there is general agreement that certain types of cases are best confined in a consultant unit where full facilities are immediately available if required. Whilst obstetric flying squads have greatly reduced the hazards of delivery in the home and in the general practitioner maternity unit with limited facilities, this is not an ideal method of dealing with complications. Where these can be foreseen it is greatly preferable that the patient should be booked for confinement in the fully equipped consultant unit, especially if, as is often the case, the latter is situated at some distance from the G.P. unit.

The generally accepted minimum standards of ante-natal care require that the patient should be seen as early as possible in her pregnancy, usually before the twelfth week, monthly thereafter until the 28th week, fortnightly until the 36th week and weekly thereafter until delivery. In many cases of course, considerably more frequent visits will be required. There are many advantages in shared ante-natal care, between doctor and midwife in domiciliary or G.P. unit cases, and between doctor, midwife and hospital clinic in cases booked for the consultant unit, but this demands the careful use of a good co-operation card carried by the patient at all her visits.

DELIVERY AT HOME

In general, the cases considered to be unsuitable for delivery at home or in the G.P. unit are:

1. Primigravidae, whose obstetric performance has not previously been tested. Not all doctors would agree with this, nor are facilities always available for their accommodation.

2. Women over 30 years of age; the rates both of complications and of maternal and perinatal deaths rise steeply after the age of 30, both in primigravidae and multiparae.

3. Women having their fifth or later child. Again both maternal and foetal risks increase sharply with higher parity.

4. Women of small stature, under 5·0 feet, who frequently have small pelves.

5. Women suffering from any medical disease such as diabetes, hypertension, heart or lung or kidney disease.

6. Women with any skeletal deformity such as fractured pelvis, scoliosis, kyphosis, old poliomyelitis, etc.

7. Women with bad obstetric history, previous abortion, still-birth, prolonged labour, instrumental delivery, post-partum haemorrhage, toxaemia.

8. Women with poor home conditions considered unsuitable for confinement, usually after inspection by district midwife or health visitor.

9. Women who are particularly nervous and apprehensive.

10. Women with marked obesity, who seem to be more liable to obstetric complications than the normal.

It has been clearly shown in a nationwide study of perinatal mortality in 1958 that where women are transferred from home to hospital when complications arise, results for both mother and child are much worse than when timely booking at the consultant clinic has been made. Early selection of the place of confinement is therefore one of the most important responsibilities of both midwives and doctors.

ANTE-NATAL CLINICS

At the first visit to the ante-natal clinic, the patient's name, address and social status are recorded, and this may indicate the need for the help of the medical social worker. Age, the duration of marriage (infertility is again likely to be associated with obstetric complication) and contraceptive practice should be determined. A menstrual history including the date of the first day of the LMP will help establish the expected date of delivery (EDD) 40 weeks or nine calendar months and seven days later. Modification for the cycle length may be required as indicated in Chapter 3. A personal medical and surgical history may point to further special investigation and treatment, and a family history regarding hereditary disease, diabetes, twinning, etc. may be relevant to the care of the present pregnancy. Finally a full obstetric history, involving all pregnancies whether completed or not, any complications of pregnancy, labour or the puerperium, the mode of delivery, the outcome for and the birth weight of any children and their present health may also be of great importance. Smoking habits should be discussed; it is clear that perinatal mortality is higher and birth weight less in infants of smokers as compared with those of non-smokers.

PROBLEMS ARISING IN PREGNANCY

The history of the present pregnancy may reveal that *sickness* has been unduly troublesome and has gone beyond the normal to the pathological, so that the patient may be vomiting all that she swallows and has become severely acidotic. The condition is described as *hyperemesis gravidarum* and is always accompanied by acetonuria. Where this does not respond to frequent small meals, glucose drinks, the avoidance of fatty or highly seasoned foods and anti-emetic drugs such as Avomine or Debendox (remember that this problem arises during the period of organogenesis and that any untried drug may cause foetal anomalies as did thalidomide), the patient must be admitted to hospital for rest, intravenous fluids and sedation until the acetonuria clears, when diet may be gradually built up again. *Bleeding* may indicate threatened abortion and if persisting may also indicate the need for bed rest and sedation. *Pain* is often due to stretching of uterine ligaments in the early months; later it may be due to red degeneration (necrobiosis) in a fibroid which is outgrowing its blood supply. Threatened abortion may be indicated by pain, and urinary tract infection, common in pregnancy (Chapter 2) should be excluded by urine culture. Acute appendicitis and other acute abdominal conditions may occur in pregnancy and may be particularly dangerous because of delay in diagnosis. Ectopic pregnancy must be considered in the early weeks and accidental ante-partum haemorrhage later. Finally, abdominal pain may be due in the latter weeks to pubic arthropathy (subluxation of the symphysis pubis—Chapter 2) or to the onset of labour. *Headache* may indicate hypertension and together with *visual disturbances* may suggest migraine, which is often aggravated by pregnancy, or the development of toxaemia. *Urinary symptoms* as we have seen (Chapter 4) are common early and late in pregnancy when they may be physiological, but here again urinary infection may be the cause.

ROUTINE INVESTIGATIONS

At the first visit, the patient's height should be measured and recorded. Blood pressure must be recorded at each visit, so that toxaemia may be recognized early (Chapter 13), and the patient should be weighed each time. Excessive weight gain is common in the obese, but in them as in those of average build may be the first indication of toxaemia. Weight loss towards the end of pregnancy may point to placental failure with diminution in the volume of liquor (oligohydramnios) which is often an indication for induction. Malnutrition is a rare cause of weight loss, in this country, but this may occur in some cases of hyperemesis. It may also be due to an anxiety state.

Examination of the urine

Examination of the urine is of the utmost importance and must be carried out at each visit.

Albuminuria is one of the cardinal signs of toxaemia (Chapter 13) but may also be due to urinary infection or to renal disease such as chronic nephritis or the nephrotic syndrome, all of them requiring special management. Finally it may be due to contamination with discharges, and if this is suspected, filtration of the urine and re-testing will probably clarify the position.

Glycosuria in pregnancy may indicate diabetes (Chapter 20) or merely a lowered renal threshold. If a significant degree of glycosuria is found and especially if it recurs, a random blood sugar estimation is indicated and if raised should be followed by a full glucose toler-ance test.

Acetonuria is found in women with severe vomiting; if it is absent, then complaints of severe vomiting are probably exaggerated. It is not uncommon in late pregnancy, but the cause of this is obscure. In the ketosis of prolonged labour, it is a clear indication for intra-venous dextrose administration.

Blood examination
Blood examination is again of the utmost importance. Firstly blood group (ABO) and rhesus status should be determined so that if post-haemorrhagic or other anaemia should require transfusion, cross-matching may be effected without delay, and so that steps may be taken to prevent, identify or treat rhesus sensitization (Chapter 17). Haemoglobin should be estimated at the first visit and if over 80 per cent (11·8G) again at 32 and 36 weeks. If it is lower, treatment and more frequent repeat examination may be required (Chapter 20). In order to eliminate as far as possible the risks of congenital syphilis, Wassermann and Kahn or other serological tests should be carried out in every pregnancy of every woman.

General examination
This should include observations of height, weight and body-build, gait and any evidence of skeletal or other deformity. One should try to form an impression of the emotional stability of the patient. Clinical examination of heart and lungs may indicate X-ray or ECG examination, or reference to a cardiologist or other physician (Chapter 20). The limbs should be examined for deformity and oedema; varicose veins tend to become much worse during pregnancy and may affect the vulva as well as the legs, causing severe discomfort. Support hose or tights may be valuable here. Dental caries is common

in pregnancy and the National Health Service has made provision
for free dental treatment for pregnant women, who should be referred
to the dentist if any abnormality is found.

Breasts

Examination of the breasts should show signs of pregnancy activity
(Chapter 4) as well as their general development. The mother should
be encouraged to breast-feed and to prepare the nipples for nursing
by massage with lanoline or one of the proprietary creams. If the
breasts are very heavy, advice about a strong supporting brassiere is
indicated.

Abdominal examination

Abdominal examination is principally concerned with confirmation
of the diagnosis of pregnancy and with assessing its duration. One
will expect to be able to palpate the uterus per abdomen in any pregnancy beyond 10 weeks, and in general the size of the uterine mass
should correspond to dates (Fig.18). If the uterus is not palpable
it may be retroverted—this may lead to abortion or retention of urine
if it persists beyond 10–11 weeks, and bimanual examination to correct this and the fitting of a pessary until about the 18th–20th week
may be required. Alternatively, the patient may not be pregnant
or missed abortion may have occurred—investigation as indicated
in Chapter 4 will usually make the position clear. This may also be
the case later in pregnancy if the uterus seems small for dates.

    If the abdominal mass is large for dates, it may be that one is
dealing with an ovarian cyst, a fibroid or some other mass and not a
pregnancy, or such a mass may co-exist with pregnancy. The pregnancy may be multiple (Chapter 9) or there may be a hydatidiform
mole, which is often larger than a normal pregnancy of equal duration. In this case, vaginal bleeding, perhaps with passage of the
characteristic chorionic vesicles, toxaemia of early onset and the
absence of foetal heart sounds on auscultation with the Sonic Aid
or Doptone apparatus will make the diagnosis clear. Perhaps the
most common cause of such a disparity is an error in the dates.

    At later visits, the progressive growth of the uterus and of the
foetus should be observed and the fundal height recorded, and compared with the expected findings in relation to the dates. The date
of quickening should be recorded, and a note of foetal movements
made at subsequent visits. The foetal heart should be auscultated at

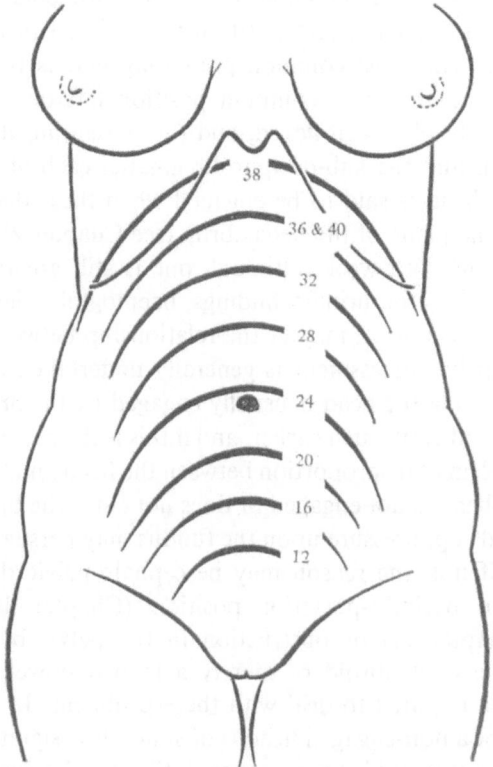

Fig.18. Fundal height at various dates.

each visit and its position noted, and any variation from a rate of 140–160 beats per minute noted. If doubt exists the Sonic Aid or its equivalent may be used.

From about the 28th week, it should be possible to palpate foetal parts with some precision. Up to about 30–32 weeks, the foetus is relatively small and the amount of liquor large, so that the position of the foetus within the uterus is quite inconstant. After this time, and as the foetus grows larger and the liquor relatively less, his position is likely to be more stable, but repeated observation is necessary to ensure that this is maintained.

The lie of the foetus describes the relationship between the foetal spine and that of the mother, and may be longitudinal, transverse or oblique. The presentation describes that part of the foetus which advances lowest into the birth canal. The position refers to the relation between the denominator of each presentation and the mother's pelvis. Each presentation has its own denominator, the occiput, sacrum or chin, and position is described in terms of this denominator. The most common presenting part is the vertex (see Chapter 2) and the most common position left occipito-anterior. With this the head is well flexed, and the presenting diameters are the biparietal and the sub-occipito-bregmatic, each of 9·5 cm (3·75 inches). The head is said to be engaged when these diameters have passed into the plane of the pelvic brim (see Chapter 2).

By about the 36th week, although one is still greatly concerned about blood pressure, urinary findings, haemoglobin levels, oedema etc., one's main concern may be the relationship between foetus and pelvis, and pelvic assessment is generally undertaken at this stage. In a primigravida the head is usually engaged by the 38th week and may be engaged very much earlier, and if this is the case it is probable that no problem of disproportion between the head and the pelvis will arise. If the head is not engaged or does not enter the brim when the patient stands up, pressure upon the fundus may persuade it to enter the pelvis. If not, the reason may be cephalo-pelvic disproportion (Chapter 9), occipito-posterior position (Chapter 10), placenta praevia (Chapter 11) or obstruction in the pelvis by an ovarian tumour, a cervical fibroid or merely a loaded bowel, and special steps may be required to deal with these problems. In a multipara, the finding of a non-engaged head is of much less significance, since in these cases it is unlikely to engage until after the onset of labour, and the previous obstetric history may show that a well-grown infant has already been delivered in a previous pregnancy.

Pelvic examination

Pelvic examination is often carried out at the first visit to the ante-natal clinic, but may be restricted at this time to cases with a special indication. All cases however should have a careful pelvic assessment at 36 weeks.

The general build and stature of the patient must be taken into consideration and any asymmetry of lower limbs noted. Vaginal examination should assess the state of the cervix (see Chapter 6) and the level of the presenting part. The diagonal conjugate may be measured by placing the tip of the middle finger upon the sacral promontory, and measuing the distance from this to the point where the index finger lies under the pubic arch. Subtraction of a factor of 2·0 cm (0·75 inches) will give a fairly accurate idea of the length of the true conjugate (Fig.19). The fingers should now be swept around the ala of the sacrum and the pelvic brim on either side, noting the concavity of the sacrum and then passing down to palpate the ischial spines and the sacro-spinous ligaments which run backwards and medially from them to the sacrum. If these will accommodate two fingers without overlap on to bone on either end, the ligament must be so long as to subtend a well-formed sacro-spinous notch, so that the pelvic cavity should be adequate for the foetus of normal size. The outlet may be assessed by placing a clenched fist between the ischial tuberosities, the patient lying on her back with knees drawn up, and by trying to fit two fingers side by side into the apex of the sub-pubic arch. If this is narrowed they will be unable to reach the apex, and this would mean that a foetal head negotiating the outlet would probably be displaced so far posteriorly as to damage the perineum (Chapter 6).

If no abnormality is found, and the presenting part fits the pelvis well, only the above clinical assessment is required, but if greater accuracy seems necessary as with a breech presentation (Chapter 10) X-ray pelvimetry may be advisable. As in the diagnosis of pregnancy, this should be deferred as late as possible in pregnancy and the mini-

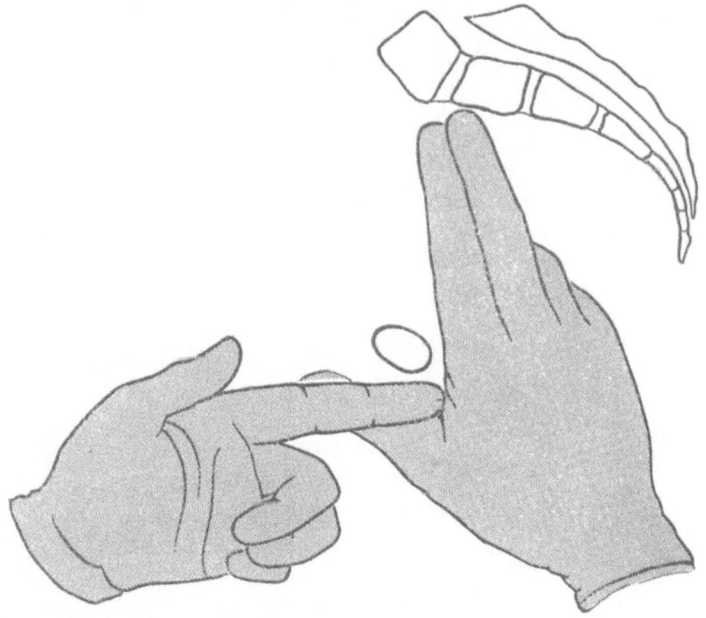

Fig.19. Measurement of the diagonal conjugate.

mal possible radiation dose used. A single lateral film will usually provide all the information required.

The attendant should be satisfied before the end of pregnancy that haemoglobin levels are satisfactory and that no abnormal feature of the pregnancy has been overlooked. Should any such feature be found, steps must be taken to deal with it as necessary.

Finally, the confidence of the patient must be gained by ensuring that she is well-received at the clinic and assured that those in attendance are interested in her well-being. In most large units now, classes in mothercraft and relaxation classes are held, whose principal value lies in informing the mother of the facts of her pregnancy and what she is to expect, whilst also ensuring that she is able to care for her baby. The full-scale programme of psycho-prophylaxis has never achieved the same popularity in this country as it has in France and Russia, but modified programmes are undoubtedly helpful to some women. Unfortunately, the women who most need such help are very often too frightened to attend, but a sympathetic interview at the ante-natal clinic may overcome this to the benefit of all concerned.

6

The physiology of labour

THE ONSET OF LABOUR

Labour may be expected to begin about 280 days after the first day of the LMP or about 266 days after conception (assuming a 28 day menstrual cycle). The cause of the onset of labour is by no means clearly understood, but a variety of factors probably play a part. There is increasing evidence that the foetus, possibly stimulated by progressive oxygen lack as the placenta ages towards term, may contribute to the initiation of labour. It is clear also that certain hormones have an oxytocic function, i.e. they cause the uterus to contract. The posterior pituitary secretes oxytocin which is destroyed by an enzyme known as oxytocinase. High levels of this enzyme during pregnancy fall away later, thus exposing the uterus to the action of oxytocin. Another inhibitory factor acting upon the uterus during pregnancy is the high level of progesterone, which acts as a relaxant of plain muscle and especially of the myometrium. When these levels fall away as the placenta diminishes its activity, this inhibition is removed and the uterus is likely to become more responsive. A further group of hormones recently discovered, the prostaglandins, has been shown to have a powerful oxytocic action when administered by various routes. Although these were originally isolated from prostatic secretions as their name indicates, they have been shown to present in various body fluids in the female. Their place in the control of normal labour however is not yet clear. Another factor which may play a part is the downward pressure of the presenting part upon the upper aspect of the cervix which by stimulation of the paracervical ganglia induces reflex contraction of the uterine body.

During pregnancy, the cervix with its sphincteric action preventing expulsion of the uterine contents is dominant, whilst the body of the uterus under the action of progesterone is quiescent. As progesterone levels fall away and other factors come into play, the roles of body and cervix are reversed, and whilst the body contracts, the cervix gives way and allows itself to be dilated by being pulled up over the presenting part. This reversal of roles however is not a sudden event since in most women the uterus is preparing for labour for as much as two months before the onset of labour proper. Throughout pregnancy, waves of activity occur in the uterus from time to time (Braxton-Hicks contractions) but these are not expulsive in character. They become more frequent towards term and may sometimes be painful, and although in the past this has been denied, they may play a part in the preparation of the uterus. In some women the cervix remains cylindrical in form, firm and tightly closed or unripe (Fig.20a), until labour is well under way. In their more fortunate sisters, the formation of upper and lower uterine segments and the effacement and early dilatation of the cervix may begin as early as the 32nd week. The myometrium like other muscles is capable of contraction, i.e. the muscle fibres become shorter and thicker and their tone increases. It also has a unique quality of retraction, whereby the muscle fibres become shorter and thicker and retain this form without increase in tone. When retraction occurs, the upper part of the uterus becomes slightly smaller and its wall much thicker as more and more of the bulk of the myometrium moves up towards

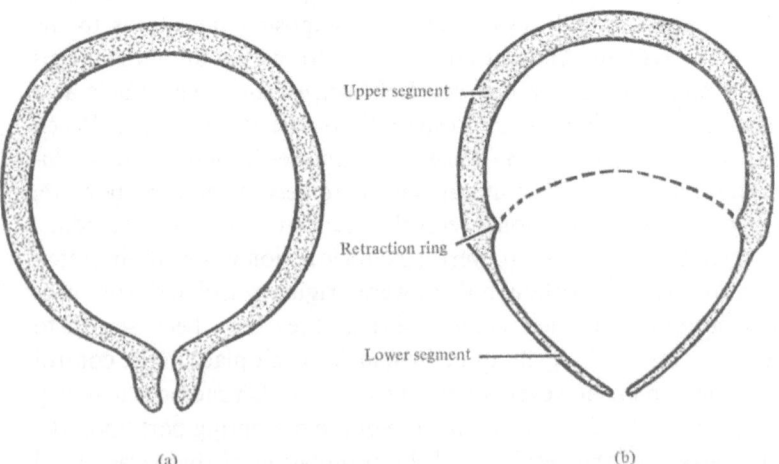

(a)   (b)

Fig.20. *a.* Unripe cervix. *b.* Ripe cervix with formation of lower segment and retraction ring.

the fundus. The remainder of the uterus, the lower uterine segment, is formed largely from the isthmus of the uterus and the cervix. In contrast to the upper segment it increases in area and becomes thinner, merging into the effaced and thinner cervix which may be as much as 3–4 cm dilated some weeks before the onset of labour proper (Fig.20b). This of course means that the work of the uterus in labour is much reduced, and in women such as this labour should be relatively easy and quick, in contrast to the generally slower and more difficult labour in the presence of an unripe cervix.

The onset of labour proper may be heralded by a 'show', a loss of blood from the vagina, usually small in amount, resulting from the separation of the membranes from the region of the internal os. Sometimes, the first sign may be rupture of the membranes, the amniotic sac giving way usually at its lowest point (the forewaters) lying in advance of the presenting part and just above the cervix. This may be confused with urinary incontinence although the opposite error is more common. A strip of litmus paper will usually serve to distinguish the alkaline liquor from the acid urine. In some cases, however, rupture of the membranes does not occur until much later in labour or even after delivery of the child, which is then said to be 'born in a caul'. An old superstition claimed that a sailor with a caul in his possession could never be drowned; no doubt on the strength of this many acres of amniotic membrane have changed hands for a suitable consideration.

Most frequently the first sign of labour is the onset of contractions or labour pains. As a rule these first appear as aching in the lower back, then later pains pass round the flanks and down towards the pubis. They are at first infrequent, recurring every 20 minutes or so, but become stronger and more frequent until they are coming regularly every 5 minutes or so. By this time labour may be regarded as well established.

THE FIRST STAGE OF LABOUR

The first stage of labour is that of dilatation of the cervix, and lasts from the onset of labour until dilatation is complete. In a primigravida this may take 8–12 hours; in a multipara the duration is usually 4–6 hours, but wide variations are found in both groups. During this stage, the uterine contractions alone represent the powers of labour. The foetus advances into the birth canal, the presenting part coming down to about mid-cavity to reach the level of the ischial spines. Over the presenting part an oedematous area forms on the scalp of the infant where the presenting part is girdled by the dilating cervix. This is the caput succedaneum and is a normal phenomenon in labour.

THE SECOND STAGE OF LABOUR

The second stage of labour is that of expulsion of the foetus and should be completed usually within an hour, but it is often much less prolonged. With full dilatation the character of the labour pains alters, and in addition to the uterine contractions, the secondary powers of labour are brought into play. The mother tends to bear down using her abdominal and pectoral muscles and her diaphragm, and she may use her limbs to obtain purchase for her expulsive effort. The change in her respiration is often noticeable and an expiratory grunt may be audible as she strains downwards. The pain becomes increasingly severe and frequent until eventually the presenting part appears at the vulva and delivery is completed. With an occipito-anterior vertex presentation (Fig.21), generally the most favourable position, the well-flexed head allows the vertex to advance to the pelvic floor. Here it impinges upon the levator of one side, and gradually, with successive pains, the occiput is rotated to the front. With further descent, the occiput emerges under the pubic arch and by a movement of flexion, the bregma, brow and face sweep across the perineum and the head is born. At this stage the longest presenting diameter is the suboccipito-frontal of 10 cm, so that stretching of the perineum should not be excessive. After its emergence, the occiput undergoes restitution to the left side and, then as the shoulders descend into the antero-posterior diameter, the head may rotate. The anterior shoulder now emerges under the pubic arch, and the trunk is born by lateral flexion.

THE THIRD STAGE OF LABOUR

The third stage of labour is that of separation and expulsion of the placenta. After delivery of the foetus, the upper uterine segment, to which the placenta is normally attached, becomes much smaller as further myometrial retraction occurs. As a result the area of placental site is greatly reduced and the placenta is sheared off. Further

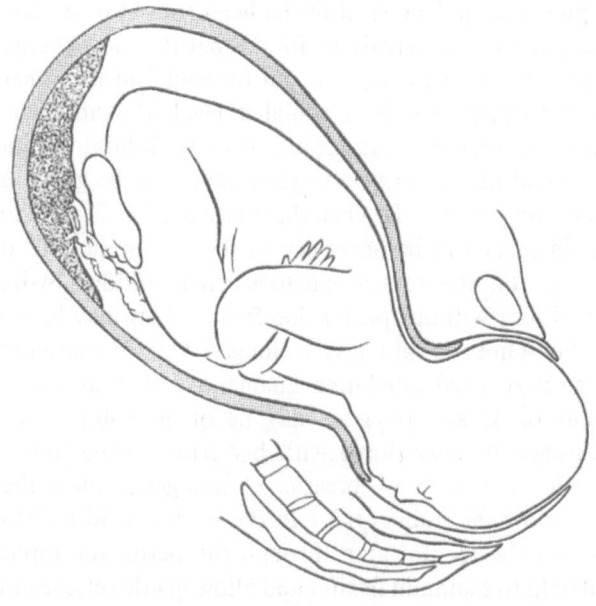

Fig.21. Delivery of head by extension: Occipito-anterior position.

uterine contraction, sometimes aided by downbearing on the part of the mother, drives the separated placenta down to the lower segment and upper vagina whence it may be easily removed. As the placenta is separated, the large maternal sinuses of the placental site are torn across; severe haemorrhage is prevented by contraction of the figure-of-eight fibres of the myometrium embracing these sinuses. The third stage is commonly completed within a few minutes, and is likely to be pathological if it lasts longer than twenty minutes.

A fourth stage of labour has been described by some authors. This is really the first hour after delivery when close observation is required to ensure that the uterus remains contracted and that no haemorrhage or other mishap occurs.

MANAGEMENT OF LABOUR

In the early part of the first stage, the patient is often very apprehensive, especially if she is a primigravida and, since the pains at this stage are not very severe, above everything she requires reassurance and sedation with promazine 50 mg, diazepam 5·0 mg or some similar preparation. The level of the head should be determined per abdomen, and it will usually be found that it is deeply engaged and well flexed so that the occiput is out of reach but the sinciput palpable on the opposite side at a higher level. If bladder and bowel are distended uterine contractions may be inhibited, and so the patient should be encouraged to pass water and be given an enema. As the first stage proceeds, when the cervix reaches 3–4 cm dilatation, better pain relief will be necessary as she will by now be distressed by her pains. It is now appropriate to give her pethidine hydrochloride 100 mg with or without promazine 50 mg. This may have to be repeated after 4 hours if labour is prolonged. Once the latter part of the first stage is reached inhalation analgesia with Entonox, a mixture of nitrous oxide and oxygen, may be of advantage. The mother is encouraged to bear down with her pains, using long expulsive efforts after a couple of breaths of analgesic, until the occiput emerges below the pubic arch and the head is said to be crowned. Pressure on the frontal area through the perineum applied with a pad will help to maintain flexion and allow gentle release of the head. If the perineum appears likely to tear, episiotomy may be carried out (see Chapter 16). The neck should be palpated to ensure that it is not surrounded by cord. If so this should be divided between clamps and disengaged. A finger placed in the anterior axilla and pulled backwards will ease the anterior shoulder below the pubic arch and then the trunk may be delivered by sweeping the shoulders forward over the pubis. The cord should be clamped doubly and divided—here 20–30 seconds delay will lead to placento-foetal transfusion and reduce the risk of respiratory distress syndrome in the newborn.

It is customary in this country to give an oxytocic injection with the delivery of the head, and either ergometrine, or syntometrine which acts more rapidly, may be used to make the uterus contract (see Chapter 21). After delivery of the child the uterus will be found extending up to the umbilicus, spherical, bulky and with limited mobility. Following the oxytocic injection, it may be expected to contract and separate the placenta. The fundus rises up to 2 finger breadths above the umbilicus and the uterine mass becomes firmer, smaller and more mobile. If it can be felt to be contracting firmly, the cord clamp may be grasped with the right hand and held firm, whilst with the left hand the uterus is pushed up and away from the placenta which may then be easily removed from the vagina (Brandt-Andrews method). This should be accompanied by very little bleeding. It is imperative that traction should not be exerted on the cord until the uterus is contracting strongly. Failure to observe this restriction may lead to inversion of the uterus which is often accompanied by severe haemorrhage and shock.

After delivery the patient should be kept under observation for the next hour, and the uterus frequently palpated to ensure that it is well contracted. The vulva should be inspected so that any lacerations may be recognized and if necessary repaired. Blood pressure should be checked—a sharp rise may occur at this stage and may presage an eclamptic fit and demand heavy sedation. A fall on the other hand might indicate unrecognized haemorrhage or some other kind of shock requiring investigation.

During this time, the foetus, now the infant, must be kept warm and comfortable, his airway must be cleared, his cord ligated or clipped to ensure that haemorrhage is avoided, and a general examination made so that any obvious congenital anomaly is recognized and any necessary arrangements made for treatment.

Careful inspection of the placenta is also important. The rough maternal surface should be examined under running water to ensure that no lobes are missing whilst the foetal surface should be checked for vessels running to its margin and there torn across, which would indicate the presence of a succenturiate lobe, a small accessory mass of placental tissue which may have been left in utero. The completeness of the membranes should also be checked.

One hour after delivery, if all seems to be well, the patient may be transferred to the lying-in ward.

7

The puerperium

The puerperium is the period following delivery usually regarded as lasting six weeks when the changes of pregnancy regress and when in some women at least, lactation is established.

After the completion of labour the uterus still remains a heavy bulky organ, the fundus lying at or near the level of the umbilicus, with a large raw area, the placental site, exposed to possible ascending infection and sometimes rather poorly drained. The vagina too has been distended and has frequently been torn, so that it too may be a portal of entry for genital tract infection. It is not surprising therefore that puerperal infection, the so-called childbed fever, has been dreaded through the ages and has caused the deaths of many hundreds of thousands of mothers. It is encouraging that with present methods of management it is rare, but meticulous attention to nursing care is essential if it is to be avoided altogether.

INVOLUTION OF THE UTERUS

Involution of the uterus and of the rest of the genital tract is the process whereby these organs return more or less to their pre-pregnant state. The remains of the decidua are shed almost as in menstruation and the remaining basal layer grows so as to cover over any raw areas. This is accompanied by vaginal discharge, the lochia, which is typically blood-stained and red for the first three days, reddish brown for the next three, and brownish or pale for a few days thereafter. The myometrium is reduced in size first of all by its contractions. In women who breast feed these are reflexly induced by suckling, and in such women the rate of involution is generally more rapid. There is degeneration and hydrolysis of many of the muscle fibres, the products of this process being eliminated via the blood-stream and lymphatics as well as in the lochia, and as a result the size of the uterus is rapidly reduced. On the first day after delivery, the fundal height is about 5 inches above the symphysis pubis; thereafter it falls by about half an inch or more (1–2 cm) daily until by the tenth day it is no longer palpable above the brim of the pelvis. Involution continues thereafter at a slower rate and is usually finally completed by about the sixth week. The vagina and the pelvic floor soon regain their tone and although the vagina remains larger than before delivery, it should be almost back to its former state in 3–4 weeks. Lacerations or episiotomies usually heal without complication if they have been carefully sutured (see Chapter 12). With the removal of relaxin the pelvic joints regain their stability, fluid being withdrawn from the joint cartilages. The abdominal muscles may have been greatly overstretched and for these as well as for the pelvic floor, remedial exercises may be of great value.

Sub-involution

Sub-involution of the uterus is often found in the grande multipara, the woman who has had 5 or more children, possibly in association with subclinical infection, but it is especially associated with either retention of part of the placenta or membranes or frank genital tract infection or both. In such cases the daily rate of involution will be slowed, the fundal height remaining at the same level for several days, and red lochia will persist beyond the expected 3 days. Inspection of the placenta and membranes after delivery may have already led one to expect this, and in these circumstances the administration of ergometrine 0·5 mg by mouth twice daily for 3 days may stimulate the uterus to expel its contents. Should this fail or should excessive bleeding occur, evacuation of the uterus should be undertaken. The os is invariably open so as to admit one finger or more, and using a modern suction curette, evacuation may be carried out without anaesthesia with little or no discomfort to the patient.

The presence of retained products of conception in the uterus particularly favours bacterial invasion, but such infection may occur even when the uterus is empty, as the placental site with its ragged decidual remnants and blood clot makes an ideal portal for entry. Infection may occur during a prolonged labour, especially with long-ruptured membranes, or may arise after delivery, from the nose, throat, or hands of attendants, from the mother's own bowel or even from the cord stump of the infant. Thirty years ago the most common and most dangerous organism was the haemolytic streptococcus; today *Staphylococcus aureus*, *Escherichia coli* and *Clostridia* are more important. Clinically the patient will present with malaise and abdominal pain, pyrexia, often an offensive lochia especially with *E. coli* infections, and tenderness and sub-involution of the uterus. In the most severe cases, the organisms may invade the blood-stream or the peritoneal cavity to produce septicaemia or peritonitis, which may be very dangerous for the patient. Commonly however, the infection is limited to the uterus, which will be found to be bulky and tender. After the collection of a high vaginal swab, the appropriate chemotherapy should be instituted and the patient and her baby isolated. If necessary the uterus should be evacuated under antibiotic cover. Most cases will respond rapidly to treatment but in some all the therapeutic resources of the infectious diseases unit may be required.

THE BREASTS

The breasts during pregnancy have been actively secreting colostrum under the control of high blood oestrogen levels, but now the oestrogen is withdrawn and a new hormone comes to the scene. This is another anterior pituitary secretion called prolactin which stimulates lactation, the production of milk. During the first three days of his life, the infant should be put regularly to the breast so that both he and the mother shall learn the techniques of suckling. The mother will benefit by more rapid involution and the infant will receive colostrum which is said to act as a laxative and help evacuate his bowel content, meconium. About the third evening there is a surge of activity; the breasts become congested and sometimes painful, occasionally with a sharp rise of temperature, and usually by the following morning all settles down and lactation is established.

In women who choose not to breast feed, restriction in fluid intake will usually be sufficient to prevent any pain or other difficulty with the breasts. The use of oestrogens to inhibit the secretion of prolactin has recently been condemned as a possible cause of puerperal thrombophlebitis and it is probably wise to avoid this completely. If pain does occur the use of a diuretic is probably all that will be required.

MENSTRUATION

Menstruation is usually suppressed during lactation, and even where artificial feeding is used, the re-establishment of menstruation is very irregular and may occur after four weeks or after several months. It should be remembered that ovulation may occur as soon as the necessary endocrine sequence is re-established and so pregnancy may occur before the return of menstruation.

THE URINARY TRACT

Retention of urine. The urinary tract may have suffered trauma during labour and bruising of the urethra is not uncommon. This together with the pain of perineal sutures may inhibit micturition, so that retention of urine may occur. This can often be recognized because of lateral displacement of the uterus, usually to the right side of the abdomen, by the distended bladder. Catheterization may be required and a careful watch should be kept for any residual retention. There is often a considerable diuresis in the first few days after delivery as the kidneys take part in the excretion of products of involution, as well as ridding the body of water retained during pregnancy, and if retention occurs, the bladder may rapidly become distended and painful.

Suppression of urine. Retention must be carefully distinguished from suppression of urine where kidney damage leads to failure of excretion of urine, and uraemia may endanger the life of the patient. This is a possible complication of several obstetric conditions and is discussed more fully in Chapter 11. This points to the importance of a careful fluid intake and output chart in the early days of the puerperium.

Urinary infection. The ureteral distension of pregnancy persists for some time after delivery and with it the risk of urinary infection. Acute episodes of pyelonephritis are not infrequent and are typically associated with sharp pyrexia, rigors and renal angle pain more often on the right side. Such cases usually respond promptly to the appropriate sulphonamide or antibiotic.

THROMBOPHLEBITIS

Thrombophlebitis is one of the constant dangers associated with pregnancy, and deaths from consequent pulmonary embolism constitute a large percentage of today's maternal mortality (see Chapter 23). The pressure of the pregnant uterus upon the large veins in the pelvis tends to slow down venous return from the legs and even the early puerperal uterus has a similar action. In women with varicose veins, or who are anaemic or who have had extensive tissue trauma during labour, there is a special predisposition to thrombosis and action should be taken to avoid these factors as far as possible. Even in the normal woman however the products of autolysis produced during involution tend to promote thrombosis, and it is important to take active steps to prevent it. For the past 25 years there has been increasing emphasis on early ambulation, most women now being up and about within 16–24 hours of delivery. Where for any reason this is impracticable active movements of the legs should be encouraged, not only by the physiotherapist but also by nursing staff. In cases especially liable to thrombosis, prophylaxis by intravenous low-molecular weight dextran has been advocated, and some have even recommended prophylactic anticoagulants. In view of the risk of haemorrhage when these drugs are used, others have preferred the use of vasodilators to promote movement of the circulation in the limbs. Superficial venous thrombosis, commonly in the internal saphenous vein, is often very painful and the application of heat may be very soothing. Deep vein thrombosis is sometimes accompanied by massive oedema of the leg, and usually carries a greater risk of embolism. In these cases, apart from vasodilators, paravertebral sympathetic block has been found valuable.

PUERPERAL PSYCHOSIS

Pregnancy and labour may impose considerable stress upon a mother, and if she suffers from any mental instability she may react to the strain with either pregnancy or puerperal psychosis, the latter in general being more common. This may express itself in various ways, but depressive illness is fairly frequent and occasional episodes of acutely maniacal behaviour may lead to violence towards the infant or to attendants. The patient often appears withdrawn, failing to respond to questions or making irrelevant answers for a day or two before the more violent manifestations appear, and should such bizarre behaviour occur it is often wise to seek the advice of a psychiatrist. Some of these patients will require transfer to a mental hospital, but in general the prognosis is good and most are discharged within a few weeks. There is a tendency to recurrence with subsequent pregnancy, and for this reason sterilization may be advisable as soon as the patient feels that she has completed her family.

It is customary today to keep mothers in hospital after delivery for 6–7 days, although many are discharged after 48 hours. If *early discharge* is to take place, it is wise to arrange prior inspection of the patient's home by the staff of the public health authority to make sure that it is suitable for the reception of a recently delivered woman and her baby, and also that the district nursing services are available to help them. Many multiparae find it advantageous to return home soon after delivery to be with their older children, and early discharge does permit more economic use of maternity beds. Certain cases are unsuitable for early discharge but it is remarkable how rarely a woman selected for early discharge has to be returned because of complications.

8

Multiple pregnancy

The term multiple pregnancy is used to describe any pregnancy with more than one foetus. Twin pregnancy is relatively common, about one in 80, but triplet pregnancy about 100 times less frequent. The higher multiples have been extremely rare until the past decade when the use of 'fertility drugs', most commonly human FSH, in women failing to ovulate has caused multiple ovulation resulting in the conception sometimes of 7 or more children.

Twin pregnancy tends to occur in families, and either mother or father may carry the tendency. Some cases are due to multiple ovulation and this produces fraternal twins which may be of unlike sex and show other differences, or from the development of two embryos in a single ovum, when the twins will be identical, alike in sex, blood groups and almost all other characteristics.

INITIAL INDICATIONS OF A TWIN PREGNANCY

A clue to the probability of twin pregnancy may be derived from the family history or from the previous obstetric history of the mother. The course of pregnancy in its early weeks is not really distinctive, but by about 20 weeks it is usually apparent that the uterus is large for dates. Not only is the fundus high but laterally the uterus is bulging out into the flanks to be spherical rather than ovoid. By the time foetal parts are palpable, it may be possible to recognize at least three foetal poles, such as two heads and a breech. Auscultation of the foetal heart at two different points is said to indicate a twin pregnancy only if two observers listening simultaneously record rates differing by at least 10 beats per minute. Hydramnios (excess of liquor amnii) is a common complication and when this occurs the abdominal mass is greatly increased and the skin often so thinned as to become almost translucent. If the diagnosis is not clear by about 28 weeks it is wise to clarify the position by X-ray. This will not only confirm or disprove the diagnosis, but will indicate the presentation and relation of the foetuses.

PROBLEMS ARISING IN A TWIN PREGNANCY

The mother carrying a twin pregnancy is subject to extra stress. Not only is there an increased demand by the two foetuses for iron and other nutrients, but the physical burden of the greatly enlarged uterus, especially if hydramnios is present, may be extremely exhausting. Two further complications of pregnancy are extremely common in these cases, namely toxaemia and premature labour. In view of all the foregoing, it has become the custom in many hospitals to admit the mothers of twins from about the 31st to the 36th week of pregnancy for rest and prevention of anaemia and other complications. This has led to greatly improved salvage of twins, since the incidence both of toxaemia and of premature labour has been much reduced. If there is no evidence of these at 36 weeks the mother is allowed home, but otherwise she may have to be kept in hospital until delivery. Frequent estimates of haemoglobin are required, and iron and other supplements given as necessary.

By means of such management one hopes to bring the mother to term in good condition, but induction may be required for toxaemia or other reasons. In almost half of all cases, both twins present by the vertex, and in about one third one by the vertex and one by the breech. Both twins present by the breech in about 8 per cent, whilst the remainder are mainly vertex or breech and transverse. Two transverse lies occur very rarely. It is hazardous to attempt to correct the position of twins, in view of the possibilities both of entanglement of the cord and of separation of the very large placental area involved.

The arrangements of chorion and amnion also vary (Fig.22). In some instances there are two placentae with two chorions and two separate amnions (dichorionic diamniotic arrangement). The chorion may be single with a single or bilobate placenta, with two separate amnions (monochorionic diamniotic) or there may be a single chorion with a common amniotic sac (monochorionic monoamniotic).

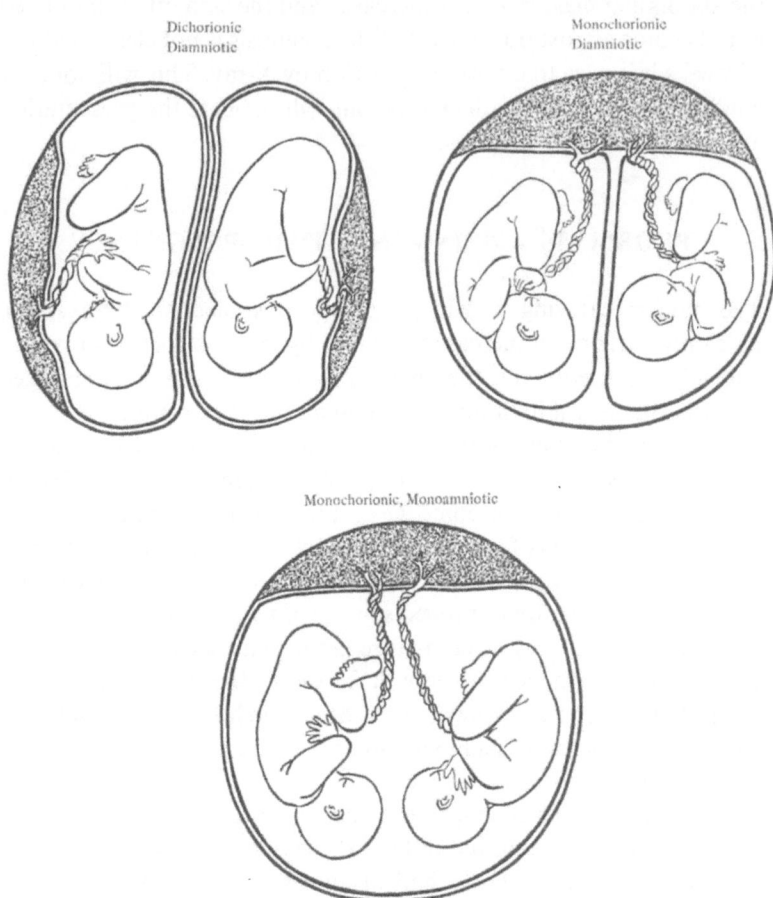

Fig.22. Various arrangements of chorion and amnion in twin pregnancy.

When labour is induced by amniotomy, it is especially important to guard against cord prolapse, particularly with the monoamniotic arrangement; indeed amniotomy is probably best avoided if possible.

LABOUR

Labour in many cases is progressive and uneventful, but especially where hydramnios is present the uterine contractions may be some-what inefficient. With the many variations of presentation, various types of manipulative delivery may be required and special problems may arise. One of these is locking of twins, where the leader presents by the breech, but the head of the second enters the pelvis as the trunk of the first comes down, and so prevents the advance of the head of the first. With general anaesthesia it is usually possible to manipulate the infants up into the uterus to free and deliver the first twin but there is considerable risk of asphyxia when the breech has been born for some time, and the manipulations may threaten to rupture the uterus. This problem however is comparatively rare, and as twins are seldom very large, cephalo-pelvic disproportion is infrequent and the first twin is usually born without difficulty. The cord should be doubly clamped and divided and the child placed in a cot (and clearly labelled Twin I). The next step is to palpate the abdomen to determine the lie, and if necessary to convert the lie to longitudinal. Vaginal examination will now show whether there is a second amniotic sac. If so, the membranes should be ruptured and the second child delivered as soon as possible. Delay may endanger the second child in view of possible cord or placental complications, and as the birth canal is already fully dilated delivery should present no difficulty. Nonetheless, the mortality of second twin is materially greater than that of first.

The third stage of labour may present problems. The placental site is much greater in area than usual whether the placenta is single or double, so that the possibility of post-partum haemorrhage is increased, particularly if one or both placentae separate before delivery of the second twin. Even after it has been emptied, the over-stretched uterus may be rather slow to contract so that atonic haemorrhage may occur. This emphasizes the importance of ensuring a good haemoglobin level during the ante-natal period; it is a useful measure to hold blood cross-matched if possible during labour of any patient with a twin pregnancy. In view of the frequent need for manipulations and for assisted delivery, the presence of an anaesthetist is also desirable.

In some instances the twins show marked differences in size. This is due not to conception in consecutive cycles (superfoetation) as has been suggested, but to the fact that the larger twin with a stronger circulation has obtained more than his share of available nutrients. In the extreme case, the development of the weaker child may be so inhibited that he remains an undeveloped mass of tissue called an acardiac monster. Sometimes the normally developed weaker child may die and be compressed against the wall of the amnion by the growth of his twin (foetus papyraceus). In a monoamniotic pregnancy, entanglement of the cords may lead to the death of one or both foetuses as the umbilical circulation is cut off.

All that has been said about twin pregnancy is true in greater degree of the higher multiples, and prolonged bed rest is essential even in triplet pregnancies. Almost all these higher multiples will suffer from toxaemia and it is rarely that such a pregnancy is carried to term. As a result, the mortality of the infants is very high indeed.

9

Pelvic contraction and deformity

THE FEMALE PELVIS

In Chapter 5 we have considered the relationship of the foetal head and the pelvis and we have studied the normal female pelvis in Chapter 2. The pelves of most women may be classified in four main groups.

1. The gynaecoid pelvis

The normal *gynaecoid pelvis*, as described above, has a well-rounded brim with the longest transverse diameter about mid-way between the sacral promontory and the symphysis, a well-curved sacrum, parallel lateral pelvic walls, and a sub-pubic angle of 90 degrees or more. This is the most favourable type of pelvis from the obstetric point of view and it occurs fortunately in over 70 per cent of women (Fig.23). A variant of the gynaecoid pelvis is the *generally contracted pelvis* whose shape is the same as that of the gynaecoid, but all of whose diameters are smaller than those detailed in Chapter 2. This type of pelvis is found predominantly in women of small stature (below 5 feet) who tend to have small children for whom the pelvis is adequate. Occasionally however they choose very large husbands for themselves, and the resultant offspring may be too large for the pelvis and demand some sort of operative delivery. On the other hand, one is often surprised at the apparent ease with which some of these small women deliver infants of 4,000G or more.

2. The android pelvis

The android, male or funnel pelvis is similar to the normal male pelvis. The brim tends to be triangular, with beaking towards the

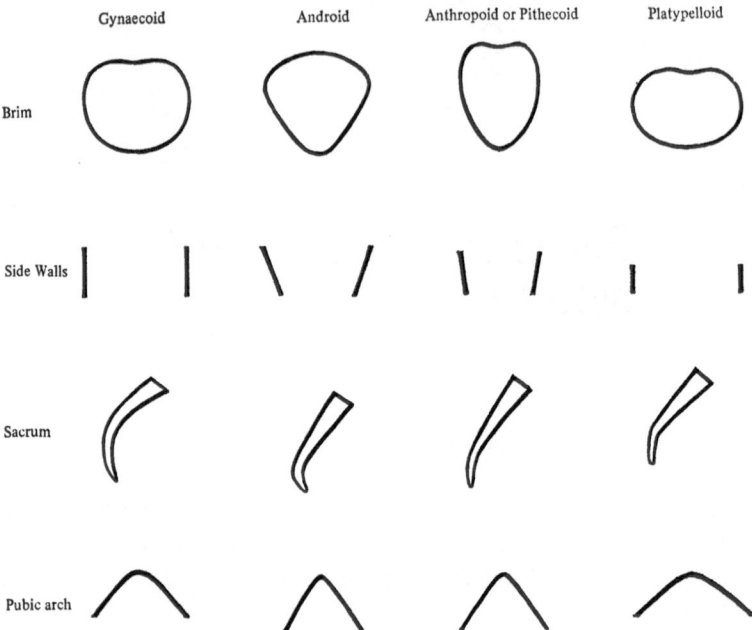

Fig.23. Features of the more common pelvic types.

symphysis and the greatest transverse diameter lying well back towards the promontory so that it is not available to the descending head. The sacrum is long and straight and tends to be inclined forward at its lower end. The side walls of the pelvis converge and the sub-pubic angle is less than a right angle. With the lesser degrees of this deformity the head may be able to negotiate the brim, only to meet increasing difficulty and become arrested as it proceeds down the birth canal so that intervention will be needed to effect delivery. Some degree of android pelvis may be found in about 10 per cent of women, and in more severe degrees it is impossible for the head to engage and Caesarean section will be required.

3. The anthropoid pelvis

The anthropoid pelvis is relatively narrow in its transverse axis at the brim, but there is usually a corresponding increase in the antero-posterior diameters. The sacrum is often straight but tends to be short and is set so far back from the symphysis that it does not seriously encroach upon the pelvic cavity. The side walls are parallel and the sub-pubic angle tends to be a little narrow. In such a pelvis, which may be found in about 10 per cent of women, an occipito-posterior head tends not to rotate to the anterior since this would involve passing through the narrow transverse diameter. Face-to-pubis delivery is therefore common and may be regarded as the most favourable available, as the long antero-posterior diameter at the outlet accommodates this mechanism adequately.

4. The platypelloid pelvis

The platypelloid or flat pelvis is found in only about 5 per cent of women. Here the antero-posterior (conjugate) diameter tends to be reduced, the transverse being correspondingly longer. The sacrum tends to be straight so that flattening involves cavity and outlet as well as brim. The side walls are parallel and set wide apart, and the sub-pubic angle is wide. This type of pelvis favours engagement with the occiput lateral, and the flat pelvis tends to inhibit rotation so that the head may become arrested on the ischial spines in this position with the head slightly deflexed (deep transverse arrest). Assisted delivery may be required, but sometimes spontaneous delivery may occur, in some instances with the occiput still lateral.

OTHER PELVIC TYPES

Apart from the foregoing a number of less frequent pelvic types may be met.

1. *The rachitic flat pelvis* formerly common in this country, is rarely seen today because of generally improved nutritional standards. In this condition forward rotation of the sacral promontory leads to flattening and difficulty at the brim; once this has been negotiated, the backward rotation of the lower sacrum permits easy delivery.

2. Following *pelvic fractures,* all sorts of bizarre shapes may be encountered, and many of these will cause cephalo-pelvic disproportion.

3. *Asymmetric pelvis* may be found in cases of unilateral disease of the lower limbs in early life, such as poliomyelitis or congenital dislocation of the hip, and whilst some of these may cause difficulty, many will permit normal vaginal delivery. Two rare developmental anomalies of the pelvis may be mentioned, in which one (*Naegele*)

or both (*Robert*) sacral alae are absent. These are usually incompatible with vaginal delivery.

4. *Spondylo-listhesis* (Fig.24), where the union of the body of the

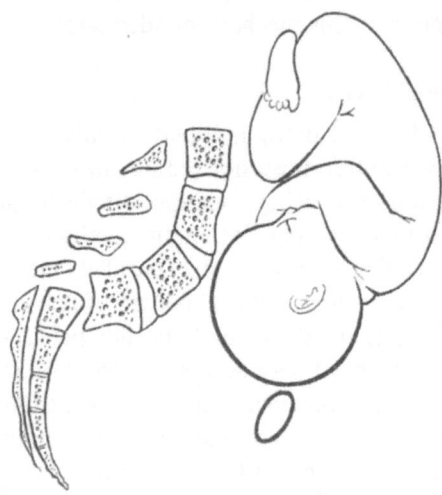

Fig.24. Spondylo-listhesis.

fifth lumbar vertebra with its arch is defective, is often complicated by a slipping forward of the body over the front of the sacral promontory. This may cause obstruction to labour, but in many instances the head can negotiate the obstacle and enter the pelvis.

5. *A wide vertebro-pelvic angle* (Fig.25) may sometimes be responsible for failure of the head to engage even in the absence of any disproportion. With the onset of labour however the head will pass down and backwards to enter the brim.

TRIAL OF LABOUR

The routine assessment of pelvic capacity at about the 36th week of pregnancy has been described in Chapter 5. It will often be obvious from early in pregnancy that vaginal delivery is unlikely; on the other hand, the outlook for delivery must always be related to the size of the child involved—in other words, the old saying, 'the foetal head is the best pelvimeter' remains true. Even with a non-engaged

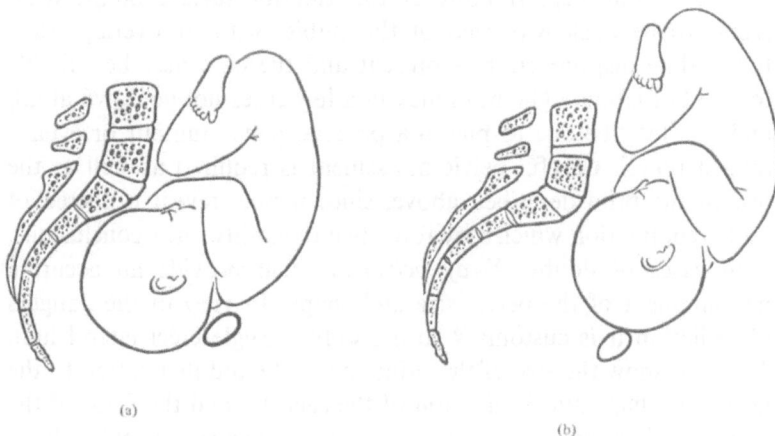

(a)

(b)

Fig.25. Vertebro-pelvic angle *a*. normal; *b*. wide

head in a primigravida at term, one may hope that with good uterine contractions moulding of the head will enable it to pass through the pelvis, and in such a case a 'trial of labour' may be decided upon. Here one tests out a variety of imponderables—the efficacy of uterine action, the degree of moulding which the head will undergo, and the effect of all this upon mother and child. The selection of a case for trial of labour requires careful judgment. Where there is obvious gross cephalo-pelvic disproportion, this is obviously unsuitable and should be treated by elective Caesarean section. Where the head, even although not engaged, can be pushed down into the pelvis no trial is needed. It is in the case with borderline disproportion so that the outcome of the trial is in some doubt that this measure is of value. In making this selection one must exclude all patients with an un-favourable obstetric or personal history or infertility, elderly primi-gravidae (today this generally means over 30 years of age) and those with malpresentation or poor emotional balance. In assessing cephalo-pelvic disproportion, a test which has been found useful is to lay the patient flat down and place three fingers of the right hand on the pubic area, the lower on the front of the pubis, the upper over the head and the middle finger over the junction between head and pelvis. If with the left hand on the fundus the head is pushed down, it may be felt to enter the brim in which case there should be no problem. If it overlaps the front of the pubis, the disproportion is so marked that vaginal delivery is highly improbable, and Caesarean section is indicated. If however the anterior surface of the head seems to lie flush with that of the pubis, without overlap, then border-line disproportion is present and the case may be suitable for trial of labour. The head may in a few cases not go down at all, and this may be due to placenta praevia, pelvic tumour or even a loaded bowel. Careful pelvic assessment is required as well as the test of the brim described above, since it may reveal a degree of outlet contraction which may force one to modify one's conclusions.

In cases of doubt, *X-ray pelvimetry* will provide an accurate measurement of the pelvic size and shape. In view of the dangers of radiation it is customary to use only a single erect lateral film. This will show the size of the brim conjugate and its relation to the head, the shape and inclination of the sacrum, and the form of the sacro-sciatic notches. In many cases of nonengagement of the head when the patient is recumbent, it will be found that on X-ray, it has been shown to have entered the brim when the patient has stood erect.

A trial of labour should never become a test of stamina between mother, baby and obstetrician, as a wise obstetrician pointed out 20 years ago. The course of labour must be watched closely and frequent observations made of maternal pulse, foetal heart and uterine action. It is probably unwise to use oxytocin to stimulate the uterus even if contractions are poor, because of the danger of rupture of the uterus (Chapter 14). Indeed, inadequate contractions may themselves be due to cephalo-pelvic disproportion. If labour is progressive and continuous increase of cervical dilatation occurs, the outlook is good. If however the cervix hangs loosely and is poorly applied to the head, the trial may well fail. One can usually reach a decision, having regard to all the facts, after 8–12 hours or even less and opt either for Caesarean section or for continuance of the trial and perhaps assisted vaginal delivery. In making this decision a standing lateral X-ray of the pelvis, which will show the level of the head, the degree of moulding and the problems still to be overcome, will be of great value. In these cases it is of course vital that strict attention be paid to relief of pain, reassurance and nutrition, probably by intravenous dextrose drip. One must never persist unduly long with a trial of labour, but so long as progress is occurring, one is justified in continuing.

10

Malpositions and malpresentations

MALPOSITIONS

Occipito-posterior positions

The most common and in general the most satisfactory presentation and position is the vertex left occipito-anterior (V.LOA). The corresponding occipito-posterior position, V.ROP, is also by no means uncommon and in the great majority of cases presents no real problem, about 90 per cent of all occipito-posterior cases being delivered spontaneously. The remainder however constitute a considerable proportion of the cases which cause anxiety, and so this malposition is of great importance. V.LOP positions are uncommon, perhaps because the rectum occupies the left posterior segment of the pelvis.

Occipito-posterior position is the most common cause of non-engagement of the head in the primigravida at term. The head is deflexed, so that the presenting antero-posterior diameter is the sub-occipito-frontal of 4 inches (10 cm).

Ante-natal diagnosis may be made by the fact that limbs may be palpable and often very prominent on both sides of the midline. The back lies in the posterior quadrant of the uterus and is not easily palpated. The head is unengaged, and deflexion can be recognized by the fact that the occiput and sinciput (brow) are palpable at about the same level. When the head is well flexed, the occiput lies at a much lower level than the sinciput. The foetal heart is usually best heard over the front of the chest, which may be thrown forward by the extension of the spine ('military position'), or over the back well out in the flank.

Manipulation to correct the occipito-posterior position at about

37–38 weeks has been advocated, but it is so seldom successful that it has largely been abandoned.

Once labour is under way, vaginal examination may show the sagittal suture running across the pelvis with the quadri-radiate anterior fontanelle palpable towards the front of the pelvis. This, as we have seen in Chapter 2, indicates not only an occipito-posterior position but also a deflexed head.

The onset of labour may be tentative because of the absence of pressure upon the cervix by the unengaged head, but once labour starts, the head usually becomes flexed and enters the brim. As a result, the more favourable suboccipito-bregmatic becomes the presenting diameter, and the vertex advances to the pelvic floor. From this point, it may undergo either long rotation through 135 degrees to occipito-anterior or short rotation through 45 degrees to direct occipito-posterior. The former is likely to be followed by normal spontaneous delivery; the latter will usually lead to delivery face to pubis, but as this commonly occurs with an anthropoid type of pelvis (Chapter 9) the end results are usually satisfactory. In about 10 per cent of cases labour will become arrested and assisted delivery be required. The occiput in these cases may remain as a persistent occipito-posterior (POP) or may have rotated to the front. In about half the cases of this group however it will become arrested with the occiput lateral, usually at the level of the ischial spines and with the deflexed head resting on the pelvic floor on *both sides* (deep transverse arrest). As a result of this, the normal mechanisms promoting rotation tend to cancel each other out and labour ceases to progress. Any of the above situations may call for assisted delivery (Chapter 16), but in some of them conservative management may lead to improved uterine activity and progress in labour will be resumed (Chapter 15). The moulding of the head in occipito-posterior positions may be characteristic, but this is not always found.

MALPRESENTATIONS

Breech presentation

This is a malpresentation since, unlike that in V.ROP, the presenting part is abnormal. The breech presents, its denominator being the sacrum, and the position is commonly left sacro-anterior, although all other variants may occur. The head will be palpable at the fundus, and ballottement may be elicited.

Breech presentation like other variations of lie and presentation is common early in pregnancy, but one can expect the foetus to adopt his ultimate situation by the 32nd–34th week as the amount of liquor becomes relatively less, and in most cases the vertex will present by this stage. As with other malpresentations, the cause of breech presentation may simply be that the head is prevented from engaging in the brim by disproportion, placenta praevia or other obstruction. Multiple pregnancy, hydramnios, poor uterine and abdominal tone especially in a grande multipara, and foetal deformity, especially hydrocephalus must be borne in mind. In many cases however no cause can be found.

DIAGNOSIS. The diagnosis of breech presentation in the ante-natal period is not usually difficult if the abdomen is always examined systematically. After inspection has confirmed the long ovoid shape of the uterine mass, the fundus should be palpated carefully, when the firm rounded head should be felt and ballottement elicited. The back and limbs should be sought by palpating both sides of the uterus and then the lower pole carefully examined. In a breech presentation one will expect to find the soft rather vaguely defined breech here; even if one has at first missed the head at the fundus, the absence of the head at the brim should send one back to look for it. After the 36th week it may be tucked away under the costal margin and especially in a well-muscled girl be easily missed. It may cause sub-costal pain and vomiting as the hard head impinges upon the ribs and the stomach, and this may afford another clue to the diagnosis. Finally, after about 32 weeks, the foetal heart is usually best heard on one or other side above the umbilicus but this is not always a reliable sign.

On vaginal examination the softer less clearly defined breech should be distinct from the harder ballottable head. In doubtful cases, radiological examination may be justified. The opportunity should be taken, by requesting a standing lateral film, of demonstrating the pelvis as well as the foetus.

The legs of the foetus in breech presentation may be flexed (*full breech*) (Fig.26b) or extended (*frank breech*) (Fig.26a) at the knees. The mass of the foetus is more rounded and the foetus more fully flexed with the former. With the latter the foetal spine is splinted and tends to be extended, and the foetal ovoid is longer so that the breech is more likely to be engaged in the brim. A variant of the full

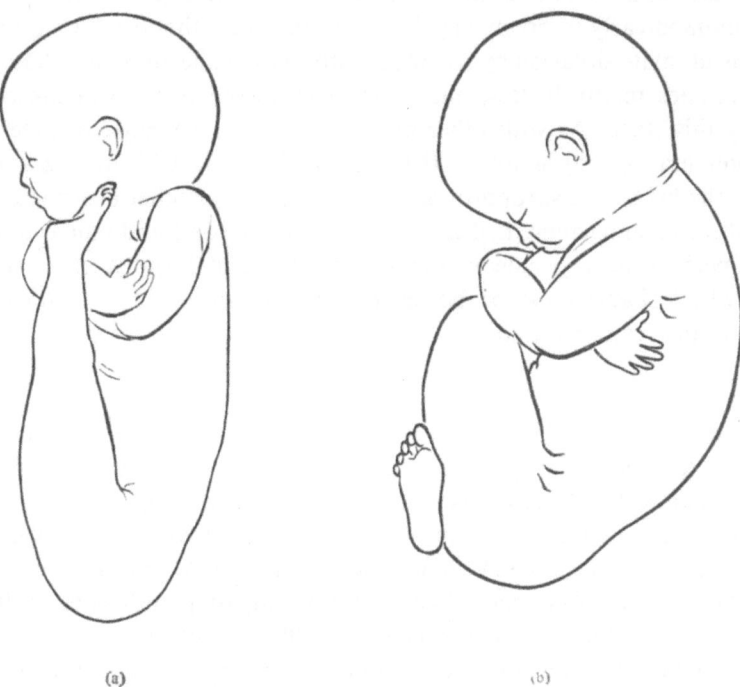

(a)   (b)

Fig.26. Attitude of foetus in breech presentation. *a*. frank breech; *b*. full breech.

breech is the *footling*, where one foot slips down below the buttocks to become the true presenting part.

EXTERNAL CEPHALIC VERSION. With cephalic presentation, the descent of the head through the pelvis occupies the whole of the first and most of the second stages of labour and moulding, if necessary, can be slow and gentle. With a breech, the body is born almost before the head enters the brim; the head must then traverse the pelvis so rapidly that the child will not inhale blood, mucus or meconium and suffer from asphyxia, and sufficiently slowly to avoid intra-cranial injury from too rapid and forceful moulding. This may present considerable difficulty and it is not surprising that the foetal mortality of vaginal breech delivery is usually 2–3 times as great as that of vertex delivery. In consequence of this, most obstetricians try to avoid the breech delivery by attempting to convert breech presentation to vertex by means of external cephalic version. This is a manoeuvre not entirely without risk. The uterus may be ruptured and so it should not be attempted after previous Caesarean section or myomectomy, and in view of the risk of placental separation it should be avoided in placenta praevia as well as in toxaemia. As we have seen in Chapter 8, there is no place for version in multiple pregnancy. Because of these risks general anaesthesia is inadvisable, and version should be persisted with only when it is easily carried out without pain for the patient. When the child is turned, the cord may be entangled, stretched or compressed, and so the foetal heart should be auscultated immediately after version. If it is found to have been seriously slowed, the foetus may have to be turned back.

Version is usually easiest about the 33rd–34th week. Before this time reversion may occur; later the increased size of the foetus and the reduction in liquor increases the difficulties. The rounder flexed breech is easier to turn than the longer extended, and engagement of the breech, commoner in the latter, constitutes another difficulty. If version is decided upon, the foetal head at the fundus should be pressed in the direction of increased flexion, whilst the breech is pushed in the opposite direction. If the uterus becomes hypertonic one should desist, perhaps to try again some days later. Even if one fails the dislodgement of the foetal position may be followed by spontaneous version. If version is achieved, one must carefully exclude disproportion or any other possible cause for the breech presentation and deal with the situation according to the findings.

BREECH DELIVERY. If version is unsuccessful, one must then decide whether vaginal breech delivery should be undertaken. Elderly primigravidae, cases with bad obstetric history, severe toxaemia or other placental deficiency, or with very large babies should be excluded. In the remainder, very careful pelvic assessment, probably including radiological pelvimetry, should be undertaken. It should be pointed out that cephalometry, measurement of the foetal skull, is not possible from an ordinary pelvimetry and only a general impression of the size of the foetus can be gained. Accurate measurement of the skull as well as of the pelvis may be made with ultrasound if this equipment is available. If any deformity or contraction of the pelvis is found, it is probably wisest to opt for delivery by Caesarean section, and this should be carried out also in those cases detailed above where vaginal delivery is contra-indicated.

In those cases that remain, arrangements should be made for

breech delivery in due course. Even now version, sometimes spontaneous, may be possible, but where this does not occur, it should
be ensured that the patient is delivered in a consultant unit. Labour
should be induced if it has not begun by term, since the increasing
size and inelasticity of the post-mature head increases the hazards.

LABOUR. The course of the first stage of labour is likely to be fairly
normal but difficulties may arise in the second stage. The limbs
and trunk in a full breech or a footling may escape through the
incompletely dilated cervix, so that the head is trapped; the frank
breech is more favourable in this respect since it is unlikely to descend
before the cervix is fully dilated. In either case, the breech will reach
the pelvic floor in due course. A caput may form on the external
genitalia, and this may lead to considerable swelling so that the
scrotum may come well down on the perineum whilst the breech
still remains in mid-cavity. In the more favourable cases, the breech
will reach the perineum with the anterior buttock under the pubic
arch. At this point the patient should be in the lithotomy position,
the perineum infiltrated with local anaesthetic or a pudendal block
carried out (see Chapter 16) and a generous episiotomy made to
facilitate any further manipulations which may be required. The
breech should be allowed to emerge from the vulva and the legs and
later the arms disengaged without traction. At this point, the head
will often pass easily and rapidly through the pelvis and delivery
will be completed without difficulty. If not, the body should be allowed
to hang down, with the back upwards, so as to bring the occiput
up against the back of the symphysis (Burns-Marshall manoeuvre).
This will promote flexion of the head which, aided by fundal pressure
from an assistant, should enter the pelvis well flexed with the sub
occipito-bregmatic and biparietal diameters presenting as in a
vertex presentation. Slight traction on the trunk which is raised
forwards and up over the mother's pubis may complete delivery.
The Mauriceau-Smellie-Veit manoeuvre (Fig.27) employs jaw
flexion and shoulder *traction*. The trunk of the child is laid along the
left forearm of the operator, the left index finger being placed in
the mouth of the infant to promote flexion. Two fingers of the right
hand are then placed at either side of the neck to exert traction
upon the shoulders. By this means, the attitude of the head may be
improved and delivery facilitated. If not forceps are applied to the
aftercoming head (Fig.28), the trunk meantime being held up by the
feet with the aid of an assistant, and delivery completed.

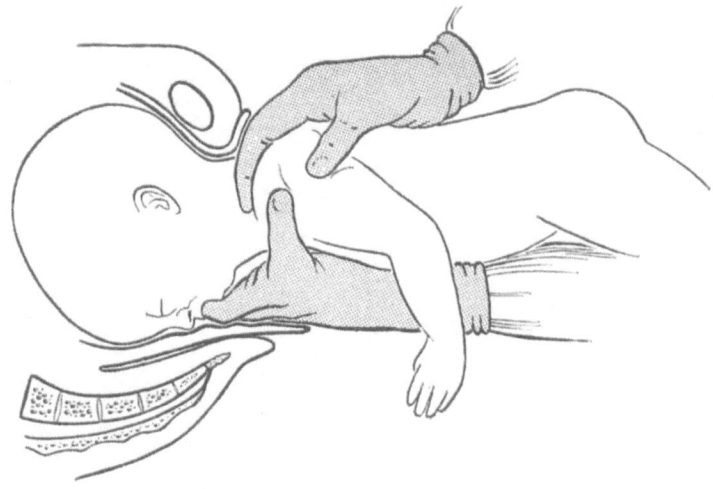

Fig.27. Mauriceau-Smellie-Veit manoeuvre.

The above as described is an assisted breech delivery and should give good results in properly selected cases. In some cases however, whether from incoordinate uterine action (Chapter 15) or unsuspected disproportion, labour is slow and tedious, the cervix may fail to dilate fully and the breech does not advance beyond mid-cavity. In such cases, there is increasing support for the view that the attempt at vaginal delivery should be abandoned and Caesarean section performed. The alternative is a breech extraction, hazardous for mother and baby and harassing for the obstetrician. Even in the best hands this operation carries a considerable mortality, and should be undertaken only by an experienced obstetrician with the aid of general anaesthesia. A detailed description would be inappropriate here.

Face presentation

Face presentation occurs when the head is fully extended, the presenting diameters being the biparietal and the submento-bregmatic and the denominator the mentum or chin. No cause is usually found; in a few cases an anterior cervical tumour or an occipital muscle spasm may be blamed.

Diagnosis may be made on abdominal palpation by feeling a large cephalic mass on one side; on the other the head cannot be reached. The back cannot be palpated until the breech impinges upon the

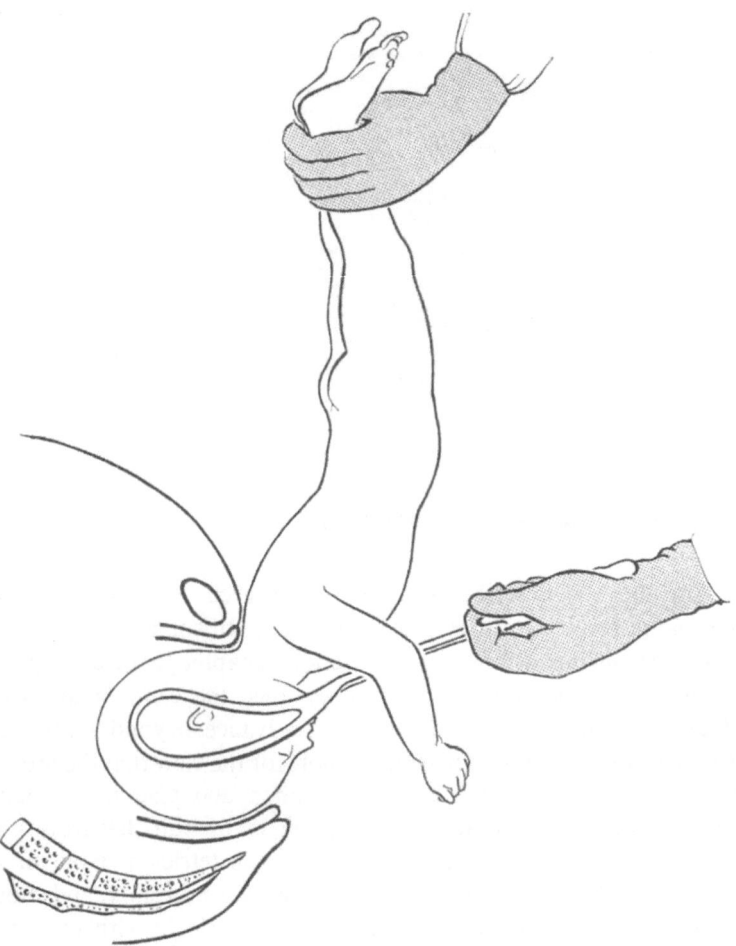

Fig.28. Forceps applied to aftercoming head.

uterine wall at the fundus. The limbs will be prominent on the opposite side and the foetal heart will be heard over the front of the chest. On vaginal examination the mouth, the nose and the orbits will be palpable, enabling confirmation of the diagnosis without difficulty. Where the chin is anterior, the mechanism is similar to that of a vertex, the chin emerging under the pubic arch and the head being born by flexion. A caput may form over the face causing bruising which may persist for some days but rarely any serious injury.

When the chin is posterior, it may become impacted in the hollow of the sacrum so that labour is arrested and rotation either by hand or with forceps will be required before delivery is possible. This however is a rare complication.

Brow presentation

The brow presents when the head is in a position midway between flexion and extension. The presenting diameter, the mento-occipital of 13·0 cm (5½ inches) is larger than any diameter of the brim and so vaginal delivery is impossible unless the presentation is modified. The only exception is when the child is very small and the pelvis very large. In these circumstances brow delivery may occasionally occur. As with face presentation, no satisfactory explanation of this malpresentation is usually found. Diagnosis is based on abdominal findings similar to those in face presentation, but on vaginal examination, the large bony mass of the brow may be felt high at the brim. On one side is the anterior fontanelle and on the other the supra-orbital ridges.

In many instances the appropriate management is by Caesarean section, but it is sometimes possible to convert the presentation to a vertex by flexion of the head under general anaesthesia. If this fails, extension may provide a face presentation. Flexion may be achieved with the ventouse re-applied further and further back towards the vertex as flexion is achieved and this may avoid the need for general anaesthesia. (Chapter 16.)

Transverse and oblique lies

Hitherto all the situations described in this chapter have referred to normal longitudinal lies. We must now consider the abnormal lies.

Transverse lies. In transverse lies the spine of the foetus lies at right angles to that of the mother, there is usually no presenting part (sometimes a shoulder may present) and no denominator. The head may lie in the right or left flank, and accordingly one refers to right or left transverse lie. There are many causes including cephalo-pelvic disproportion, placenta praevia, pelvic tumours etc. Two other causes however play a larger part in transverse lie than in the conditions considered above, namely anomalies of uterine development and lack of abdominal and uterine tone so that the lie is completely unstable and may vary from one minute to the next.

Diagnosis is usually easy. Inspection of the abdomen will show the wide transverse diameter of the uterus. On palpation the head will be felt, and may be ballotted, at one side and the breech at the other. No presenting part is palpable at the brim. On vaginal examination no presenting part can usually be reached, but late in labour the shoulder or the ribs may be palpable. In the neglected case the appearance of the hand at the vulva may finally indicate the diagnosis.

If the patient goes into labour, there is a strong risk of prolapse of the cord when the membranes rupture, and in this case emergency Caesarean section is likely to be required. Alternatively, the shoulder may become impacted in the brim, so that the overstretched lower uterine segment may rupture, and if manipulations such as internal version are attempted this danger is increased. (In internal version, the hand is introduced into the uterus to grasp the feet, bring the breech down into the pelvis and deliver by breech extraction. It is a hazardous and virtually obsolete manoeuvre.)

From the foregoing it is obvious that correction of a transverse lie is essential before labour begins. Version may be easy, especially in the unstable group, but so too is reversion. If it is repeated weekly until the foetus is large enough to maintain his position this may sometimes solve the problem, but, even if the forewaters are ruptured and drained, whilst an assistant holds the head in the brim to prevent cord prolapse, the transverse lie may recur. The patient should be instructed to report at once should there be any sign of labour, or may even be admitted to await its onset. Version may not be possible especially in cases of uterine anomaly, and in these circumstances abdominal delivery is essential. Where a longitudinal lie can be maintained in labour, vaginal delivery should be possible, but when transverse lie persists or recurs during labour, Caesarean section should be carried out. When this has been necessary in one pregnancy, repeat section will almost certainly be required in the next.

Oblique lies. In oblique lies, either the head or the breech may lie in one or other iliac fossa (oblique cephalic or oblique breech). There is no true presenting part, the head or the breech often being displaced from the brim by placenta praevia or some other mass. Other causes similar to those causing transverse lie may also operate here. In the absence of an obstructing mass an oblique lie may often be pushed over so that the now presenting part may be made to engage. Rupture of the forewaters is less likely to be followed by reversion and so vaginal delivery is more probable than with transverse lie. Caesarean section may however prove necessary, because of either placenta praevia or cephalo-pelvic disproportion and the threat of cord prolapse remains.

11

Ante-partum haemorrhage

Ante-partum haemorrhage is defined as bleeding from the genital tract after the 28th week of pregnancy and before delivery of the child. It may be accidental, inevitable or incidental, i.e. it may be due to premature separation of the normally situated placenta, to placenta praevia or to some local lesion of the lower genital tract. To consider the last group first, the lesion may be in the cervix and may range from a vascular erosion or a polyp to a carcinoma each of which demands its own treatment or even none at all.

PREMATURE SEPARATION OF THE NORMALLY SITUATED PLACENTA, ABRUPTIO PLACENTAE, ACCIDENTAL HAEMORRHAGE

This condition may be associated with pregnancy toxaemia, hypertension or trauma as from external version or a road traffic accident. It is claimed that it is due to lack of folic acid but a recent prospective study of a very large group of women treated with folic acid as a prophylactic found no reduction in incidence in the test group as compared with controls.

Bleeding may be concealed, revealed or mixed. In the first, the haemorrhage is retro-placental and no external bleeding occurs. In revealed haemorrhage, the blood escapes from the placental margin and tracks down to the cervix between the membranes and the uterine wall, and thence to the exterior. The majority of cases are mixed, showing both types of haemorrhage. When blood accumulates behind the placenta it causes severe irritation and spasm of the overlying myometrium. This may cause severe pain and shock disproportionate to the amount of blood loss. Sometimes the blood will track through the bundles of myometrial fibres and reach the peritoneal surface. As a result the uterus becomes blackish in colour —the Couvelaire uterus.

Occasionally there is a small warning haemorrhage, but usually the first appearance of the condition is a massive haemorrhage. A predisposing cause may have been present, but often no such cause is found. The patient is frequently severely shocked, with hypotension and rapid feeble pulse, and the foetus may become so hypoxic that no foetal heart is audible on admission. The uterus is woody, hard and very tender, especially if the placenta is anterior, and the patient may complain of severe pain. Vaginal bleeding may or may not be present.

Treatment of shock with powerful analgesics, morphine 15 mg or Omnopon 20 mg and blood transfusion is usually the first step. If the foetal heart is still audible, Caesarean section may be required, but in a multipara or if labour has begun and dilatation of the cervix is under way, rupture of the membranes should be carried out as soon as possible. This will reduce the tension inside the uterus and relieve pain and shock, as well as interrupting the harmful stimuli proceeding towards the kidney. As soon as delivery is possible, it is wise to empty the uterus and either the ventouse or the forceps may be used as appropriate. In the third stage of labour, as the placenta is already partly separated, post-partum haemorrhage may be a problem (see Chapter 12). The bright red blood of post-partum haemorrhage is easily distinguished from the black retro-placental clot due to the primary ante-partum haemorrhage.

Complications

Two major complications of accidental haemorrhage must be borne in mind.

1. Firstly, a shut-down of the afferent glomerular vessels of the kidney may occur and lead to *renal cortical necrosis*. This tendency is reduced by prompt amniotomy but it is wise to keep an indwelling catheter in the bladder and to check hourly urinary output. If it falls below 15 ml per hour, paravertebral sympathetic block with a local anaesthetic may interrupt the pathway of noxious stimuli from the uterus. The tendency is towards recovery, but in order to limit the dangers to the patient from uraemia, dialysis may be required and early transfer to a renal unit advisable. So long as a

satisfactory urinary output can be maintained and if biochemical monitoring gives no cause for anxiety, prompt recovery may be confidently expected.

2. The second major complication which arises in association with accidental haemorrhage is concerned with disturbances of blood-clotting. For some years, this has been attributed to hypofibrinogen-aemia resulting from intravascular clotting in the region of the damaged retro-placental myometrium. It has been postulated that the damaged tissues in this area have produced thromboplastins which have depleted fibrinogen from the circulating blood so that clotting is impossible, and uncontrollable post-partum bleeding may ensue unless fibrinogen replacement is undertaken. This may be effected by giving triple strength plasma or pure fibrinogen. More recently, it has been suggested that the administration of heparin will liberate fibrinogen from the areas of intravascular clotting. Another problem in this field is that of fibrinolysis, in which existing clots may be lysed by substances called fibrinolysins; this may be overcome by the administration of epsilon-amino-caproic acid (EACA). Clinically, the existence of this type of problem may be recognized by the obser-vation of failure of shed blood to clot, or of resolution of clots which have previously formed. A simple side-room test, Fibrindex, may indicate whether or not fibrinogen deficiency exists, but more sophisticated laboratory tests for serum fibrinogen may be necessary.

PLACENTA PRAEVIA

In placenta praevia, the placenta is situated wholly or partly in the lower uterine segment. It will be remembered (Chapter 6) that the lower uterine segment expands from as early as the 32nd week or even earlier. This leads to detachment of that part of the placenta which is attached to the lower segment and to consequent bleeding. Four degrees of placenta praevia are recognized (Fig.29). In grade 1, only the lower margin encroaches upon the lower segment; in grade 2 it reaches to the edge of but does not cover the os; in grade 3, the os is completely covered, but the margin of the placenta does not extend far beyond it; in grade 4, the placenta lies wholly in the lower segment, its margins extending well away from the os in all directions. The extent of separation, and the amount of blood loss increase with

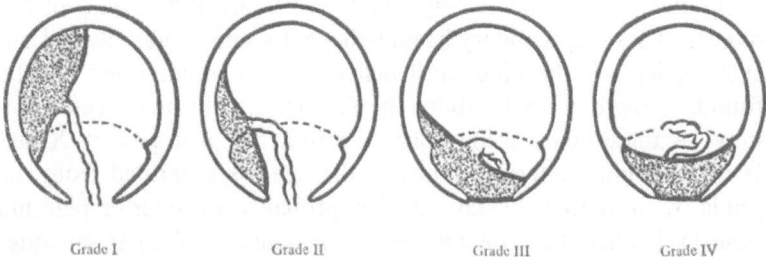

Grade I   Grade II   Grade III   Grade IV

Fig.29. Degrees of placenta praevia.

each grade, and the higher the grade, the earlier in pregnancy symptoms are likely to appear. The condition is more common in multiparae but no adequate explanation of the cause of placenta praevia has ever been put forward.

Unlike the situation in accidental haemorrhage, the bleeding in placenta praevia is painless, causeless and recurrent. There is no uterine spasm and no pain. The patient often wakes from sleep to find that she has been bleeding and no trauma or other cause is recognized. Although the first bleed is usually a small warning haemorrhage, more severe losses may follow later.

On admission, the condition of the patient is usually excellent. The uterus is relaxed and there is no abdominal tenderness. The lie and presentation of the foetus are almost always abnormal, and transverse and oblique lie and breech presentation are common. The head, if it presents, lies high above the brim and may be deviated to one or other iliac fossa. The foetal heart is usually strong and regular but as bleeding commonly occurs 6–8 weeks before term, delivery should be postponed if possible. *There is no place for vaginal examination* in such a patient until she has reached 38 weeks and is fully anaesthetized in an operating theatre, with all arrangements made for immediate Caesarean section if required, since even gentle palpation may give rise to torrential haemorrhage.

The patient should be sedated, anaemia corrected if necessary and cross-matched blood held in readiness for transfusion lest a further haemorrhage, which may be much more severe, should occur. In the absence of such a haemorrhage, the aim should be to bring her to the 38th week and to undertake definitive treatment at that stage, so as to anticipate the further haemorrhage which will almost certainly take place if she approaches closer to term. Meantime, if bleeding has ceased, she may be allowed up after a few days. In some units, such patients may be allowed home, but in view of the danger of severe secondary haemorrhage it seems preferable to keep such patients in hospital until delivery if accommodation can be found. If there is doubt about the diagnosis, placental localization may be undertaken using sonar, radio-active isotopes or X-ray. If in a standing lateral pelvimetry the head is separated from the pubis by more than 2·5 cm, there is probably an anterior placenta praevia; if when the patient is semi-recumbent a similar gap separates the head from the sacral promontory, a posterior placenta praevia is likely. The greater the gap, generally speaking, the greater the degree of placenta praevia.

At 38 weeks or earlier if one's hand is forced by recurrent haemorrhage, the patient is taken to theatre and anaesthetized. If there is little doubt that there is a marked degree of placenta praevia, or if there is a breech or an abnormal lie, it is probably best to proceed at once to Caesarean section. If the vertex presents and it is thought that the placenta praevia is grade 1 or anterior grade 2, then examination under anaesthesia may be appropriate, and if one's opinion is confirmed, amniotomy with a view to later vaginal delivery may be carried out. If a placenta praevia of grade 2 posterior, which would be compressed against the sacrum by the descending head, or of grade 3 or 4 is recognized, then Caesarean section is essential.

Problems may arise during operation if the placenta is anterior, and some authors have advocated a classical vertical incision near the fundus to avoid the placenta. This however, is unnecessary if one extracts the child without delay even if one's incision has to pass right through the placenta and the lower segment incision is almost always preferable (see Chapter 16).

If vaginal delivery occurs, the same problem may arise in the third stage as with accidental haemorrhage, namely that the placenta is already partially separated and the stage set for post-partum haemorrhage. In most cases, however, the complete separation and expulsion of the placenta is soon achieved, and bleeding controlled.

12

Post-partum haemorrhage

As we have seen in Chapter 6, the control of bleeding in the third stage of labour depends upon prompt separation and expulsion of the placenta, followed by firm uterine contraction to control the maternal blood sinuses of the placental site. This mechanism may fail for a variety of reasons, and lead to post-partum haemorrhage which may often be so severe as to threaten the life of the mother. By definition it is described as a blood loss of 500 ml or more, or such lesser amount as seriously to endanger the well-being of a woman who for example was previously anaemic. This complication has cost the lives of many thousands of women, although today with improved management and the better facilities provided by increased hospital confinement and the prevention or treatment of pregnancy anaemia, the risk is greatly reduced.

Trouble may arise when the placenta is partially separated, but not completely free and so retained. If no separation occurs a material degree of bleeding is unlikely, but partial separation, while exposing some of the sinuses of the placental site, will interfere with their control by preventing adequate uterine contraction. This partial separation may occur in cases of ante-partum haemorrhage (Chapter 11) in some cases of incoordinate uterine action (Chapter 15) and especially with bicornuate uterus, where a contraction ring may form across the base of one cornu and incarcerate the upper part of the placenta (Fig.30). It may also be found in cases of uterine scarring following Caesarean section, myomectomy or deep curettage. *Placenta accreta* is a condition where the placenta is morbidly adherent because of deep chorionic invasion of the decidua and into the myometrium. If, as one frequently finds, this is partial, the normally adherent part will become detached but the remainder will be firmly fixed to the uterine wall. Placental attachment over a myoma may be abnormal, and as the myoma cannot contract, separation may not take place. In all of these circumstances, haemorrhage may occur more or less severely.

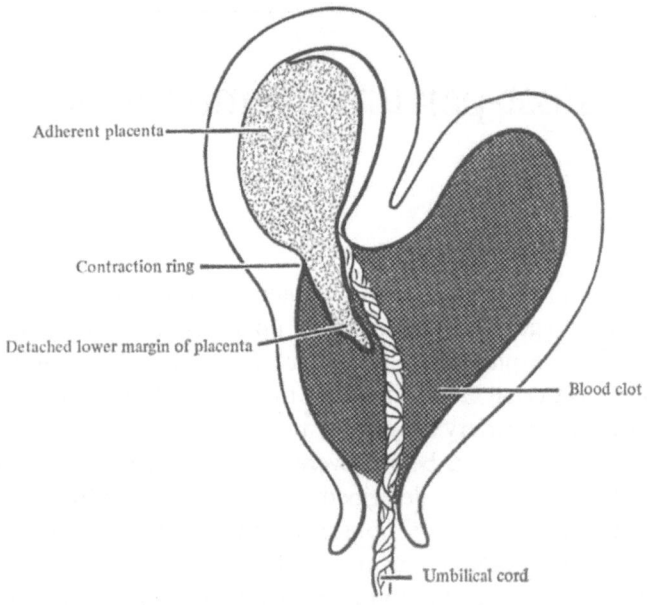

Fig.30. Placenta retained by contraction ring in bicornuate uterus.

MANAGEMENT OF POST-PARTUM HAEMORRHAGE

The management of such a case requires prompt action by both midwife and obstetrician. If the bladder is full this may interfere with uterine contraction, and following catheterization the placenta may be rapidly expelled. If the patient has become shocked, the use of morphine 15 mg will prevent further deterioration until definitive treatment can be completed. A further injection of an oxytocic drug may help the uterus to contract so as to limit blood loss. If an intravenous drip is set up, oxytocin may be given by this route. Blood replacement is of course essential to combat shock. Ultimately however control of bleeding will depend upon evacuation of the placenta, and this may be possible by a Brandt-Andrews manoeuvre (Chapter 6). If not, manual removal of the placenta will be required.

Whilst general anaesthesia is desirable, in an emergency it may be performed without anaesthesia, and if for any reason no other help is available and severe bleeding continues, it may have to be undertaken by the midwife. The gloved right hand is inserted into the uterus to seek the plane of cleavage between placenta and uterine wall, whilst the left hand upon the fundus presses it down towards the internal hand. By means of a gentle sawing motion the placenta is freed right up to the fundus and removed. If a contraction ring is present, the administration of amyl nitrite by inhalation from a 'brisette' will cause it to relax and allow access to the upper part of the uterus. Further oxytocin will now ensure that the uterus contracts actively, and once resuscitation is complete the patient may be sedated and transferred to the lying-in ward. As a working rule it is wise to aim at raising the blood pressure to 100 mm Hg or more before undertaking manual removal, but bleeding may be so severe that it is expedient to proceed before this has been achieved.

In those cases where the placenta remains adherent and there is no blood loss, simple manual removal as above should be carried out as soon as possible. Even in the absence of blood loss, retained placenta may cause shock after some hours. As observed in Chapter 6, if the third stage lasts longer than 20 minutes it is wise to take steps to ensure prompt removal of the placenta.

The obstetric flying squads

The obstetric flying squads now established all over the country were originally set up to deal with obstetric emergencies in the home, and post-partum haemorrhage and retained placenta have always been the most frequent reason for calls. The woman who has suffered a severe haemorrhage travels very badly, and shock may be aggravated to a lethal degree if the patient is moved to hospital. If she is resuscitated and dealt with on the spot, she may be moved safely or transfer may prove unnecessary. The decrease in domiciliary confinement together with better selection of high risk cases for hospital has greatly reduced the number of calls to the home, but to some extent, these have been replaced by calls to G.P. units.

The midwife who has difficulty in obtaining medical aid in the patient's home is entitled to summon the flying squad if, in her opinion, continued bleeding is endangering the patient. The squad should comprise obstetrician, anaesthetist and midwife and their equipment should include blood and saline with giving sets, sterile clothing, catheters and suture instruments as well as anaesthetic equipment and a wide range of drugs, so that even in the patient's home, management similar to that in hospital may be undertaken.

UTERINE ATONY

Some cases of post-partum haemorrhage occur after the removal of the placenta owing to failure of the atonic uterus to contract. This may be due to exhaustion after a long and incoordinate labour, or may follow delivery under general anaesthesia. It will usually respond promptly to oxytocics, but as an emergency measure, *bimanual compression* of the uterus may allow time for these to act. In the presence of very severe bleeding the uterus is compressed between a fist in the anterior fornix and the other hand pressing down from the abdomen.

Some cases where bleeding has been thought to be due to uterine atony, are in fact due to *retained placental fragments*, and routine careful inspection of the placenta and membranes should reveal that this may have happened (Chapter 6). Bleeding may occur at once or may be delayed as much as six weeks, when *late post-partum haemorrhage* may sometimes be severe. In some cases oral ergometrine may be helpful, but where there is bleeding prompt evacuation should be carried out.

TRAUMATIC POST-PARTUM HAEMORRHAGE

Traumatic post-partum haemorrhage is generally due to injury to the cervix or to the lower genital tract. In such a case after removal of the placenta the uterus may be felt per abdomen to be well-contracted, but bleeding from the vagina persists. Delivery may have been quite normal but precipitate delivery or instrumental intervention may have been undertaken. A cervical tear is commonly found on one or other side, and may extend right up across the lateral fornix to involve the uterine artery. A formal repair under general anaesthesia with full surgical facilities is necessary and care must be taken that the ureter is undamaged. Severe bleeding may also come from vaginal, vulval or perineal lacerations, especially in the region of the clitoris, and not only accurate repair but blood transfusion and other resuscitative measures may be required.

RUPTURE OF THE UTERUS

It is important after any delivery to palpate the uterus from time to time to ensure that it is not filling up unnoticed with blood. Similar occult bleeding may occur into the base of the broad ligament if the uterus has ruptured, and the insidious development of shock in such cases may be followed by sudden extreme collapse. So-called 'silent' rupture of the uterus may occur after an apparently normal delivery in a grande multipara, but often some predisposing cause such as previous uterine perforation or Caesarean section or manipulations such as internal version will have taken place. In any case where possible rupture of the uterus is suspected, exploration under anaesthesia is essential so that repair or even hysterectomy may be carried out if indicated.

13

Toxaemia of pregnancy

This condition, also called pre-eclampsia or pre-eclamptic toxaemia, less satisfactory descriptions as eclampsia follows infrequently, is peculiar to pregnancy and is characterized by hypertension, oedema and albuminuria, one or more of which may be present in the individual case. It is commonly found in the last trimester of pregnancy, but rarely it occurs earlier, especially in association with hydatidiform mole. Its aetiology is unknown, but it is more common in primigravidae and in association with multiple pregnancy, hydramnios and diabetes. It appears to be quite distinct from essential hypertension, but some degree of pregnancy toxaemia is frequently superimposed upon this equally poorly understood condition.

The basic problem here, although the aetiology is not understood, appears to be that the mother may be threatened by a variety of possible disastrous complications, including eclampsia, accidental haemorrhage, renal failure and cerebral haemorrhage. The foetus too is at risk, since toxaemia is associated with damage to the placenta, retardation of foetal growth and possible intra-uterine death.

In the absence of any known cause for this condition many theories have been put forward, but none has yet been shown to provide the true answer. In the light of the increased incidence of toxaemia in primigravidae, in multiple pregnancy and in hydramnios, all of them conditions associated with increased intra-uterine pressure, the utero-renal reflex theory of Sophian and Franklin has a certain appeal. They believe that the increase in tension within the uterus gives rise to stimuli which in turn lead to renal vasospasm and thence to the recognized manifestations of toxaemia. It is generally agreed that there is a reduction of flow not only in the renal cortical circulation but also in placental, hepatic and possibly the cerebral circulation, and it is striking that in cases of toxaemia, amniotomy with release of intra-uterine tension is commonly followed by a fall in blood pressure.

The reduction in placental blood flow leads to a parallel reduction in the supply of oxygen, nutrients, hormones and other products of placental metabolism to the foetus, and the resultant impairment of growth gives rise to a small-for-dates foetus; if the deprivation becomes severe, this may lead to foetal death.

DIAGNOSIS

No unquestionable criteria for the diagnosis are available as the aetiology is not understood, and so this must be based upon meticulous observation of the patient during the ante-natal period.

As we have seen in Chapter 5, routine observation of the blood pressure will show a considerable range in different women, but a significant rise in the individual woman must be seriously regarded. On the other hand, when a woman presents with a raised blood pressure late in pregnancy and the previous levels are unknown, it is difficult to assess its importance. This is one reason why it is desirable that the obstetrician should see his patient as early as possible in pregnancy so as to be able to compare late and early findings. Again, records of weight gain throughout pregnancy will afford a far greater insight into what goes on than a single measurement when pregnancy is already well advanced.

The successful management of toxaemia must depend upon early diagnosis and this in turn must rely upon meticulous attention to the detail of ante-natal care. The first clue is usually a rise in blood pressure and some excess weight gain may be observed before any oedema is clinically recognizable. Albuminuria is usually a late sign but in a few cases may be the first to appear.

Blood pressure. The upper limit of normal blood pressure is about 130/90 mm Hg, but in women whose normal pressure is low a rise to a lower figure may be significant. The systolic pressure may be very labile in response to stress or emotion and may to some extent be disregarded, but a rise in the diastolic is always significant.

Weight gain during pregnancy is normally around 26 lbs (12 Kg) and in the later weeks of pregnancy should not exceed 1¼lbs (0·5Kg) weekly. A figure higher than this will usually be found associated with some degree of *oedema*, at first in the feet and legs, later in abdomen, hands and face. It is often demonstrable first over the medial (sub-cutaneous) surface of the tibia above the ankle, and may be very gross. Tightness of the rings is obvious when the hands are swollen, but loss of facial contours may be recognized only following diuresis after delivery.

Albuminuria. When albuminuria is found, one must try to exclude causes other than toxaemia including contamination, infection and pre-existing renal disease by filtration, culture and microscopy respectively, but albuminuria appearing for the first time late in pregnancy is most commonly due to toxaemia.

Associated symptoms and signs may appear in the more severe cases. Headache is common and may be due not only to hypertension but also to cerebral oedema. Eye signs include blurring of vision, double vision, scotomata (loss of part of the visual fields) and even temporary blindness, due mainly to papilloedema (swelling of the optic disc). Vomiting may occur as a result of increased intra-cranial pressure. Epigastric pain is associated with congestive changes in the liver. Oliguria may appear as renal function is progressively impaired. All these together with tremors and twitching are classed as signs of imminent eclampsia, and may presage the onset of a fit.

Tests of renal function are of little value in diagnosis apart from the measurement of urinary output and of albuminuria. The blood urea is commonly low, about 18–20 mg per cent, possibly due to fluid retention. The measurement of serum proteins may show a reduction in total proteins, with reversal of the albumin-globulin ratio in the more severe cases, as albumin leaks into the renal tubules whilst the larger globulin molecule is retained. The daily variation in the albumin content of the urine may usefully be measured with the old fashioned Esbach albuminimeter, which, although admittedly inaccurate, provides sufficient precision for clinical control.

TREATMENT

Bed rest. The great cornerstone of treatment is bed rest, and in all but the mildest cases this should be undertaken in hospital. It has been generally observed that patients suffering from toxaemia do less well at home, and may show progressive deterioration which is reversed when they are transferred, perhaps because of more complete separation from family cares. Recumbency appears to be associated with improved placental and renal blood flow, with consequently better foetal growth and increased urine output. The latter may amount to a considerable diuresis after the first 24 hours or so of bed rest with regression or disappearance of oedema, relief of headache and of eye signs etc.

Diuretics. There is some disagreement about the value of *diuretics*, but if oedema is slow to disappear the use of such preparations as chlorthalidone or frusemide two or three times weekly may be justified.

Hypotensive agents may be of value where the blood pressure is very high (diastolic over 110 mm Hg) and rauwolfia alkaloids including reserpine, although their hypotensive activity is small, may be potentiated by diuretics, and have a valuable secondary effect in promoting improved renal blood flow.

Sedatives are widely used in this condition and such preparations as phenobarbitone, diazepam, amylobarbitone and promazine may be of value, although their use is occasionally complicated by the appearance of drug rashes.

After an initial phase of complete bed rest, the mother may be allowed up at first for toilet purposes only and later more freely; if all her signs and symptoms regress she may be allowed home to continue rest there, but she will require close supervision by her general practitioner and district midwife and should be recalled in a week or so to the ante-natal clinic for review, in case re-admission is required.

During her stay in hospital, apart from the usual routine observations she should have blood pressure checked twice daily, albuminuria if any measured daily, foetal heart auscultated twice daily, weight measured weekly, haemoglobin estimated weekly and such other tests as are considered necessary. Any deterioration in blood pressure or urine output must be reported, and if the former should rise to a very high level 4-hourly or more frequent recording may be desirable.

The infant is of course at risk from progressive placental failure, which is often poorly related to the apparent clinical severity of the toxaemia, extensive infarction sometimes being found even in mild cases, especially if the disease has begun relatively early in pregnancy.

EXAMINATION OF FOETUS

The foetus must be examined frequently to assess its size, and to observe whether it is growing. Clinical estimation can only be approximate, but today sonar offers a very accurate means of measuring the growth of the foetal head and *serial cephalometry*, carried out weekly has given useful results. *Urinary oestriol* estimations, usually on a 24 hour urine, give a valuable indication of the metabolism of the foetus since the oestriol excreted by the mother is largely derived from foetal suprarenal activity. Serial estimations carried out weekly or more often should show a progressive rise as pregnancy approaches term. A fall indicates that the foetus is in danger as does a range below the average for the period of pregnancy. Toxaemia, with its associated placental damage, is one of the most common causes of the *'small-for-dates' or dysmature baby* (see Chapter 19). The placenta suffers progressive fibrosis and infarction, and its various functions become increasingly deficient so that the child is deprived of oxygen and nutrients and the hormones produced by the placenta fall to sub-normal levels. This not only threatens the growth of the foetus but may lead to intra-uterine death, and so *induction of premature labour* is one of the most important methods of management available. As the pregnancy approaches term the normal pre-term placental senescence is super-added to the toxaemia, and the combined result may seriously threaten the foetus after the 38th week. For this reason, induction of labour at 38 weeks is advised almost as a routine. Even if the foetus remains rather small, this is probably due to dysmaturity and continuation of the pregnancy is unlikely to lead to further increase in size whilst it may seriously reduce the prospects of survival. In more severe cases of course, worsening of the signs and symptoms of toxaemia as well as increasingly unfavourable foetal findings may indicate earlier induction, and it may be desirable to terminate pregnancy as early as the 32nd week. In such cases, the outlook for the child is necessarily poor, but continued pregnancy may be even more lethal. If the child's condition seems particularly critical, delivery by Caesarean section may sometimes offer a better chance; this avoids the inhibition of placental blood flow and compression of the foetus during uterine contractions which in such a case may be fatal.

COMPLICATIONS OF TOXAEMIA

In most cases, the measures described above enable one to bring the pregnancy to 38 weeks before termination is required. In some however early intervention may be required in the interests of the foetus. In others intervention may be required because of deterioration in the condition of the mother, in order to anticipate and prevent the serious complications which may ensue if it is allowed to progress too far.

Eclampsia. Continued rise of blood pressure to very high levels, increasing albuminuria with diminished urine output, headache, visual symptoms and vomiting have been described above as indicating imminent eclampsia.

Premature separation of the placenta. This is true in certain cases, but in others who escape eclampsia, the disorder progresses to premature separation of the placenta or accidental haemorrhage (Chapter 10).

Renal cortical necrosis with oliguria and anuria going on to uraemia may follow as a further consequence of either of the above conditions or may result merely from progressive deterioration in the toxaemia itself.

Acute hepatic necrosis. A rare but highly dangerous complication is acute hepatic necrosis, which may be heralded by intractable vomiting and severe epigastric pain with progressive jaundice and ketosis. This may sometimes be reversible with parenteral dextrose and insulin therapy, and here the cooperation in treatment of a physician is of the first importance.

Cerebral vascular accidents. In the presence of severe hypertension it is not surprising that cerebral vascular accidents may occur. These may be found in association with aneurysm of the circle of Willis, but intra-cerebral bleeding may also occur. The prognosis is usually good, but permanent neurological damage may result.

In all the above conditions prompt termination of the pregnancy is essential. The child may be already dead, but if not there is a limited place for Caesarean section. In most cases however amniotomy followed by an oxytocin drip is the method of choice, and in these cases, as in the labours of all patients suffering from toxaemia, assisted delivery should be undertaken as soon as practicable. Maternal efforts to bear down in the second stage must be discouraged as they may lead to further damage.

ECLAMPSIA

This is a condition of convulsions arising in a pregnant woman usually following upon a worsening toxaemia, but occasionally arising de novo in an apparently normal pregnancy. The convulsions may be single or multiple, and in the most severe cases may be virtually continuous, the so-called status eclampticus. Eclampsia may be ante-partum, intra-partum or post-partum, according to whether fits occur before, during or after labour.

The fit usually begins with a tonic stage when the patient becomes rigid, holds her breath, becomes cyanosed and loses consciousness. This may last for about a minute, and may be complicated by pulmonary oedema, acute heart failure or acute hypoxia which may lead to the death of the foetus. This stage is followed by the clonic stage which commonly lasts 2–3 minutes with violent convulsive movements during which the patient may injure herself. This in turn is followed by gradual recovery of consciousness in the favourable case, and by a variable interval after which another fit may occur. The more rapid and complete the recovery of consciousness, the fewer the fits, and the longer the interval between fits the better the outlook. Prolonged unconsciousness with failure of recovery between fits and frequent and numerous fits indicate an unfavourable prognosis. It is useful to catheterize the bladder; if several hundred millilitres of urine are obtained, the underlying renal condition is still good and the prognosis better than if little or no urine is found.

Treatment

Treatment of eclampsia is primarily prophylactic, and in countries with good ante-natal care the incidence of eclampsia has fallen to a very low level. Early recognition and treatment of toxaemia and timely interruption of pregnancy have largely contributed to this. In some countries, eclampsia is less common than it might be because of malnutrition, and there was a striking reduction of the frequency of eclampsia for the same reason in Holland during the German occupation in 1942–3. In Australia it has been claimed that eclampsia can be abolished if the weight-gain during the second trimester is limited to not more than 8 lbs (4 Kg).

Diagnosis is not usually a problem. The convulsions in epilepsy are very similar, but usually a history of this condition may be obtained from either the patient or her friends; other causes of fits in late pregnancy are rare.

Even where signs of imminent eclampsia have developed it may still be avoided by timely termination of pregnancy and heavy sedation. Phenobarbitone sodium 200 mg by intramuscular injection has been found useful for this purpose, especially in cases with a sharp rise of blood pressure post-partum. A more recent introduction is chlormethiazole edisylate (Heminevrin) which may be given by intravenous drip when a fit is thought to be impending, when its anti-convulsant action may be of great value.

Once convulsions are present, one's first responsibility is to treat the fits. It is important to maintain an airway and to prevent the patient from injuring herself. Oxygen should be given by mask to limit the maternal cyanosis and the foetal hypoxia and heavy sedation administered to prevent further fits. Phenobarbitone sodium or morphine may be given if the patient is not in hospital and she should be transferred immediately. On arrival, more effective sedation may be achieved with bromethol, freshly prepared in a dose relative to the estimated weight of the patient and placed in the patient's rectum as a low-volume enema of 60–100 ml. As an alternative an intravenous drip of thiopentone sodium may be used, and adjusted so as to keep the patient lightly unconscious; it may be accelerated if a further fit threatens. A second alternative is the use of a lytic cocktail of pethidine 100 mg, promethazine hydrochloride 10 mg, and chlorpromazine 25 mg, by slow intravenous injection. In this situation also there may be a place for chlormethiazole, and diazepam is also being used increasingly frequently,

As a result of these measures, the patient should be kept lightly unconscious for several hours during which she must be constantly supervised and her airway maintained and oxygen administered as necessary. Strong lights or noise may stimulate further fits, and she should be kept in a darkened room as quiet as possible. Further examinations made at this point should include catheterization of the bladder (see above) and obstetric assessment. If the child is alive, there may be a place for Caesarean section, but if the cervix is favourable or if the foetal heart is absent, induction by amniotomy and intravenous oxytocin is usually preferable. Delivery should be assisted with the ventouse or forceps as soon as practicable.

Once the uterus is empty there is usually rapid improvement, but moderate sedation should be maintained for 24–48 hours, and urine output carefully watched in case of renal complications. The eclamptic patient is commonly grossly oedematous and a vigorous diuresis may be expected during the early days of the puerperium. In post-partum eclampsia, the sedative measures described above will usually bring fits rapidly under control. Once a good renal function is re-established, blood pressure will usually fall quite rapidly and in most cases albuminuria will clear within a week. In the few cases in which raised blood pressure and albuminuria persist, the question must arise whether in fact one is dealing with a chronic nephritis. It may be difficult to decide upon this for three months or more, since by this time all signs and symptoms of toxaemia will certainly have gone whilst those of nephritis will persist.

The *outlook for future pregnancies* is usually good. Where a first pregnancy has been affected, the next may escape altogether or the toxaemia may be mild. Only in the worst cases is recurrent toxaemia likely to be severe. In one group however, the situation may get worse with each successive pregnancy. In the older patient who has escaped toxaemia with her first three or four pregnancies, but who suffers fairly severe toxaemia with a late one, the problem is likely to get worse with each successive pregnancy, possibly owing to functional ageing of her viscera. In such a case, sterilization may well be advised.

The results of pregnancy in cases with *chronic nephritis* are in the main discouraging, with a high foetal mortality and a considerable risk of an unfavourable effect upon renal function. Careful assessment of each case must be made as in some it may be wise to advise termination.

In women with *essential hypertension* the course of pregnancy may be quite normal, but many are complicated by superimposed toxaemia when the course is similar to that of an uncomplicated toxaemia. In some instances the blood pressure will fall during pregnancy but may rise in the puerperium to unprecedented levels and cause anxiety. It will usually settle back to its previous level after six weeks or so.

14

Induction of labour

INDICATIONS FOR INDUCTION

Induction of labour, where steps are taken to persuade the uterus to contract and so expel its contents, is being used increasingly all over the world and in some obstetric departments as many as 40–50 per cent of all patients are treated in this way. The most common indications are found in a variety of situations in which the well-being of the foetus is threatened by further continuance of the pregnancy, and induction may be employed before term, at term or when the pregnancy has proceeded beyond the expected date of delivery. In some instances the induction is indicated in the interests of the mother rather than of the foetus.

A large range of indications for induction may be quoted. Of these perhaps the most common are toxaemia and postmaturity. The former is discussed in Chapter 13, and other indications for induction of premature labour include some cases of rhesus sensitization (Chapter 17) and some of unstable lie (Chapter 10). In foetal malformation and intra-uterine death of the foetus, premature induction may save the mother from weeks of unprofitable continuance of her pregnancy, and in the latter group may spare her from the dangers of clotting defect sometimes found in association with retention of a dead foetus in utero. In diabetes and in other situations where premature placental failure may threaten intra-uterine death in the last weeks of pregnancy, induction may make possible a greatly improved foetal salvage.

Postmaturity is associated with increased foetal risk because of the progressive deterioration in placental function which begins some time before term and continues beyond. It has been shown that the risk to the child is increased fourfold after the 42nd week as compared with that in the 38th–40th week. This risk increases with maternal age, and so it is commonly advised that induction should be undertaken about ten days after the estimated date of delivery (EDD); in women over 30 induction within a day or two of EDD is recommended. In some women indeed, in whom in a previous pregnancy intra-uterine death has occurred before term and has been attributed to *placental insufficiency,* premature induction at 38 weeks or even earlier has given good results.

Induction may also be undertaken in a few cases where painful uterine contractions occur for some weeks before term, or where necrobiosis in a fibroid causes pain. In addition there are many individual cases in which induction may be considered advisable; so called 'elective induction' for social or fiscal reasons is widely practised in some parts of the world.

In any case in which induction is contemplated, the growth and maturity of the child must be carefully considered so that the risk of producing a premature child incapable of survival may be avoided as far as possible. The accuracy of the patient's dates must be studied and a review of the ante-natal records made to reconsider fundal heights, date of quickening etc. It is notoriously difficult to estimate accurately the size of the child, but if it seems to be very small, one must consider whether it would not benefit from some further weeks of intra-uterine growth. On the other hand, small size of the child may be due to placental failure, and if, on the basis of urinary oestriol levels or other findings, it is considered that the risks of continued stay in utero would outweigh those of prematurity, induction should be proceeded with.

In reaching a decision on this point, apart from biochemical monitoring *amnioscopy* may be helpful. By this means, the forewaters are inspected by passing a lighted conical tube through the cervical canal. If the liquor is clear or white (from flakes of *vernix caseosa,* waxy material desquamated from the skin of the foetus) it may be reasonable to defer induction until repeated serial amnioscopy shows a greenish discolouration due to meconium staining (see Chapter 19).

METHODS OF INDUCTION

Two main methods are in general use, surgical and medical.

Surgical induction

Surgical induction in the past has comprised the introduction of foreign bodies of various kinds into the lower uterine segment, so as to stimulate labour by irritation of the uterus. Because of the risks of infection these have been entirely abandoned in favour of *amniotomy* (rupture of the membranes). Because it was believed that the dilating effect of the bag of forewaters was vitally important, hindwater rupture with a Drew-Smythe catheter used to be the favourite method. This is an S-shaped metal cannula with a stilette which may be advanced to project beyond the tip. The cannula is introduced between the membranes and the uterine wall, the stilette advanced, and as much liquor as desired drawn off. Since the value of the forewaters has been questioned, this method is used only for certain special indications, such as the placing of an intra-amniotic catheter for the monitoring of uterine activity. Instead, forewater rupture is carried out using curved or straight Kocher's forceps or amniotomes expressly designed for this purpose, and in general results are better. One must beware of the possibility of cord prolapse, and sometimes the operator may find the cord already lying in the forewaters below the head (*funic presentation*). In such a case it is wise to desist and have recourse to Caesarean section. Following amniotomy, the state of the liquor should be noted; yellow discolouration may indicate rhesus sensitization, greenish liquor is usually meconium-stained indicating foetal distress, clear or turbid liquor is normal. Some estimate of the amount of liquor may also be helpful. If it is markedly reduced (oligo-hydramnios) this usually indicates deterioration of the amniotic cells, which is commonly accompanied by impaired placental function. Any of these signs will demand especially careful monitoring of the foetal heart.

Following amniotomy, one may expect labour to be established in over 75 per cent of cases within 24 hours. The results tend to be less satisfactory in grande multiparae and in women in whom the cervix is unripe and the lower segment poorly formed. For this reason, it may be helpful to use a preliminary 'ripening' oxytocin induction on the day before amniotomy; after this, even if labour has not been successfully induced, the cervix may be more favourable so that the prospects of success with amniotomy are enhanced.

Rupture of the membranes may expose the patient and her baby to the risk of ascending infection so that she may suffer a metritis and her child an intra-uterine pneumonia which may prove lethal before or after delivery. The risk is increased as the interval grows longer between amniotomy and delivery, and for this reason it is advisable to use prophylactic antibiotic cover with such preparations as cephaloridine, which has been shown to cross the placental barrier, in cases undelivered after 24 hours.

Medical induction

A variety of drugs acting upon the uterus has been used in attempted induction, but most of these have been discarded as being either ineffectual or dangerous. The response of the uterus to oxytocic drugs varies from woman to woman, and even from hour to hour in the same woman, so that dosage must always be tentative and adjusted according to the uterine response. If uterine hypertonicity is induced it carries for the mother the risk of possible rupture of the uterus; the foetus is at risk because of the interference with placental blood-flow which uterine spasm will cause. Medical induction must always remain therefore under continual supervision by trained personnel and should be undertaken only in hospital where full facilities are available for all necessary treatment.

The OBE method. The OBE (castor-oil, bath and enema), the traditional medical induction of the midwife, should be discarded as an archaic and ineffectual cruelty to the mother. The castor oil acts as an irritant to the bowel, and any associated stimulant action upon the uterus is so slight as not to justify the unpleasantness of the medication. The bath has hygiene to commend it, and the enema, by promoting evacuation of a loaded bowel, may clear the way for labour, and these two procedures retain their value.

Use of oxytocics. Quinine and other drugs have long been discarded as toxic to the foetus and today the only oxytocics widely used for induction are *posterior pituitary oxytocin* or more commonly one of its synthetic equivalents, Pitocin or Syntocinon, and more recently the prostaglandins (see Chapter 6). The last are now generally available, and current research suggests that they may be found valuable for the induction of labour.

The place of oxytocin in the initiation and control of normal labour has recently been questioned but there is no doubt that its administration for induction will lead in most women to uterine contraction. Intramuscular administration has been used in the past, but has recently been condemned because if hypertonicity does occur, the drug cannot be withdrawn. Administration by intranasal spray may be helpful in the promotion of lactation but is unsuitable for induction. As a result, the only routes used today are intravenous and buccal. In the former an intravenous drip of 5 per cent dextrose is set up containing 1–5 units of oxytocin per 500 ml, and the drip begun at a low rate (10–15 drops per minute) and doubled every 30 minutes until a uterine response is obtained. Once pains are established and coming regularly every 3–5 minutes the drip may be switched off, to be resumed if uterine activity falls off. If hypertonic contractions should appear the drip should again be switched off and the intensity of contractions may be expected to fall away by 50 per cent within 15 minutes. In all cases the drip rate should be adjusted in accordance with the uterine response, and the half-hour gap before it is increased is necessary since it may be thirty minutes before the full response is elicited to any particular dosage level.

As an alternative method of administration the placing of tablets in the upper buccal sulcus may be used. The available tablets contain 200 units of oxytocin, and are scored so that 100 units may be administered. Smaller tablets of 50 units will soon be on the market, and this will facilitate the use of lower dose schedules. Although the required dosages are very much higher than with intravenous administration, the effect is measured in the same way, and dosage built up in accordance with the uterine response. This principle of oxytocin titration until satisfactory uterine activity occurs has been described by Turnbull in respect of intravenous therapy, but it may be used equally well with buccal oxytocin. Additional tablets are placed in the mouth at half hour intervals (just as with intravenous therapy) so as to build up to an effective dosage; if an excessive response occurs, it can be reduced by 50 per cent in 15 minutes by removing the tablets and washing out the mouth (exactly as with the drip). Buccal administration avoids some of the discomforts and risks of intravenous therapy and in particular avoids the overloading with water which might be dangerous in some cases of toxaemia, especially since oxytocin itself has an anti-diuretic action. The objection that absorption is less regular than from the drip may be true, but is of little importance if the principle is accepted that dosage must be determined in accordance with uterine response. Oxytocin must be regarded as a dangerous drug, whatever the route of administration, and its safe employment must depend upon meticulous supervision of its effects.

With the ordinary methods of intravenous or buccal administration of oxytocin a high success rate is to be expected, with about 97–98 per cent of patients in labour within 40–48 hours from amniotomy. The results are much less satisfactory without preliminary amniotomy, and a shorter induction delivery interval will be obtained if oxytocin is administered within an hour or two of rupture of the membranes.

A refinement in the administration of oxytocin has been provided by the Cardiff Oxytocin Infusion Apparatus, whereby a carefully measured dose of from 1–32 milliunits per minute may be given by means of an electric pump. The rate of flow may be adjusted electronically by means of an intra-amniotic cannula so that the dose of oxytocin will be set by the strength of uterine contractions. With this apparatus, failure of induction should be completely eliminated, and the problem of the patient who is still not in labour 48 hours after amniotomy should no longer arise.

Using the ordinary methods of administration it is customary to measure duration of induction from the time of amniotomy. If the patient is not in labour after 12–18 hours, a first drip or a first $4\frac{1}{2}$–5 hour buccal course of oxytocin is given. If labour does not ensue, a second drip or a second course is given after 24 hours; if at the end of this time, 40–48 hours after amniotomy, labour is not established it is usual to undertake Caesarean section in 2–3 per cent remaining. It is to be hoped that the Cardiff Apparatus will obviate the need for this by overcoming with safety the problem of the unresponsive uterus.

15

Incoordinate uterine action

As we have seen in Chapter 6, the uterus during labour acts as a dual organ, that is the upper segment is contracting and somewhat reducing its size whilst the cervix is permitting itself to be dilated and the lower uterine segment undergoing stretching and thinning, which may begin several weeks before the onset of labour. If polarity between upper and lower segments is satisfactory, labour is likely to be easy, swift and progressive. If on the other hand, the reciprocity between the two segments is defective, the uterine action is said to be incoordinate and labour may be long, difficult and tedious.

There are many predisposing factors. Tension and anxiety, especially in the young, the old and the unmarried primigravida may express itself in spasm of the lower segment, and much of the value of ante-natal relaxation classes lies in overcoming this problem. It is helpful too if the patient is given every opportunity to become familiar with the place where her baby will be delivered and with the people who will look after her, long before labour begins.

Apart from psychological causes, the elderly patient may have physical changes in the uterus, and the presence of fibroids may interfere with contractions. During involution after each pregnancy, a proportion of the muscle fibres of the myometrium are replaced by fibrous and elastic tissue, and in the grande multipara this will often result in inefficient uterine action, so that the woman who has had a number of children 'like shelling peas' finds herself to her outraged dismay having a long and difficult labour. Local disease or operation upon the cervix, such as a Manchester operation or even cauterization may rob it of its elasticity and interfere with dilatation. In some cases, the cervix seems to contract pari passu with the body, and this may lead to a very painful and quite unprogressive type of labour—the so-called cervical dystocia.

Where the presenting part fits snugly into the pelvis as in V.LOA positions, the reflex stimulation of the upper segment by the pressure of the hard head upon the cervix is likely to elicit powerful contractions. Where this is not the case, as in occipito-posterior positions and malpresentations as well as in cases of cephalo-pelvic disproportion, the response of the upper segment is likely to be much less satisfactory. In some of these cases there is failure of formation of the lower uterine segment, so that the cervix remains unripe and the conical lower part of the uterus of itself tends to prevent descent of the presenting part.

In all the above situations, the onset of labour may be slow and irregular and infrequent pains may continue for many hours. Contractions tend to be shortlived but none the less may be very painful, and severe backache may occur particularly with occipito-posterior positions or cases with the cervix lying towards the posterior fornix (sacral position of the cervix). Pains may go on for many hours without apparent change in the state of the cervix so that the patient becomes exhausted and acidotic, with dehydration, vomiting and acetonuria. The foetus too may suffer as a result of prolongation of labour and develop signs of foetal distress.

MANAGEMENT OF INCOORDINATE UTERINE ACTION

If the doctor or midwife can gain the full confidence of the patient, this may go far to prevent incoordinate action in the tense and frightened group. A kindly reception both ante-natally and at the onset of labour with sedation as required and later analgesia when pains become more severe will be well repaid. Simple physical treatment, such as ensuring that bladder and bowel are empty, may greatly enhance uterine action.

When the condition is already established and a tired and frightened woman is admitted, the most important thing for her is rest and nutrition. The former may be obtained by using a powerful analgesic such as Omnopon 20 mg (which seems to be much more effective than pethidine or pentazocine in this situation) so that she may rest between pains and possibly sleep if only for an hour or so. It is remarkable how in some such cases, the mother wakes up greatly refreshed, the whole character of the labour changes to become more progressive, and she goes on to deliver herself or at least to reach a stage where assisted delivery may be undertaken. At the same time, intravenous dextrose 5 per cent should be given and the drip continued until delivery. Oral feeding is best avoided because of the increased probability in these cases that anaesthesia may later be required for Caesarean section, with possible exposure of the mother to the risk of Mendleson's syndrome (Chapter 23).

Causes of incoordinate uterine action

Incoordinate uterine action should not be taken at its face value and every effort should be made to determine its cause.

1. *Cephalo-pelvic disproportion* must be excluded; this is to be suspected if the presenting part remains high, and if on vaginal examination, the cervix is found hanging loosely and poorly applied to the presenting part. As we have seen (Chapter 9) this may be so gross as to indicate immediate Caesarean section. In less severe cases, improved uterine action may effect sufficient moulding of the head to attain delivery, and a standing lateral intra-partum X-ray pelvimetry may help one to make the decision as to whether this is likely. If the head is fully engaged and moulding not too marked, in the absence of outlet contraction one can hope for a successful outcome. Pain relief and a little rest, with correction of acidosis, may be all that is required but if this proves ineffectual a short trial of stimulation of the uterus with a closely supervised oxytocin drip may be justified. This however must be rigorously excluded if disproportion is more than very slight.

2. *Hypertonicity of the uterus.* In some cases, hypertonicity of the uterus may occur, especially if it has been overstimulated with oxytocin, but it may also arise spontaneously. General hypertonicity is characterized by continuous pain with no relief; the uterus on palpation feels continuously hard with no softening between pains as in normal labour. This leads to rapid exhaustion of both mother and foetus, and if prompt vaginal delivery cannot be effected, Caesarean section is required. Localised hypertonicity occurs as constriction ring. In normal labour, the junction between upper and lower segments is marked by a *physiological retraction ring* which during labour rises up to a point a little above the level of the symphysis pubis. In contracted pelvis and other cases of obstructed labour, the *pathological retraction ring* (Bandl) rises to a much higher level in the abdomen as the upper segment continues to contract

powerfully in its efforts to overcome the obstruction. The lower segment is meantime stretched and thinned progressively until it may rupture. The physiological retraction ring may be palpable on the inner surface of the uterus but not per abdomen. *Bundl's ring* may both be seen and palpated as a transverse depression rising higher and higher in the uterus, and is an indication for urgent action to empty the uterus before rupture occurs. It must be distinguished from *constriction ring*, a localized area of contraction which may occur without obstruction during the third as well as the first and second stages of labour. It represents a special form of incoordinate uterine action and leads to arrest of progress in labour. An area of 'hour-glass' contraction may be recognized around some narrower part of the foetus which does not relax when the rest of the uterus does so. In the third stage, as we have seen in Chapter 12, it may grasp the placenta, commonly in a bicornuate but often in a normally developed uterus. Attempts at delivery of either foetus or placenta may be unsuccessful until the ring can be made to relax, either with deep general anaesthesia or more simply and safely by the inhalation of amyl nitrite.

Incoordinate uterine action may often be successfully managed by the means described above, but in a proportion of cases treatment will fail, and intervention of some kind will be called for. The exact indication may be prolonged labour or maternal or foetal distress, but in a majority of cases incoordinate uterine action will be the underlying cause.

PROLONGED LABOUR

It has been shown that results are poor for both mother and child in cases where labour is prolonged beyond 24 hours. In the past, the risks of intervention were so great that ultra-conservative attitudes prevailed and labour was continued for many days. As better techniques were evolved, nutrition was improved, and haemorrhage and infection were better understood and managed, attitudes have changed and it is today far more dangerous to temporise and allow labour to go on too long than to intervene in good time. In a patient not already in a consultant unit who is not nearing delivery after 15–18 hours of labour it is probably wise to transfer her to the better equipped unit for further management.

MATERNAL DISTRESS

This is usually easy to recognize. The mother will become increasingly tired, anxious and depressed as labour proceeds. Temperature and pulse may rise, and dry tongue and sweet-smelling breath may indicate dehydration and ketosis. Dilatation of the large bowel may be recognized in some cases as exhaustion increases. Uterine contractions may be weak or strong, but the mother becomes more and more distressed by them, even with apparently adequate analgesia, and begs her attendants to 'do something', a request which should rarely be refused.

FOETAL DISTRESS

The classical signs of foetal distress are:

1. *Variation in the foetal heart rate* from the usual 140–160 beats per minute. At first it may tend to become more rapid, but later slowing is more significant and it may fall to 80 or less. Irregularity is also to be noted especially during uterine contractions and this becomes more significant if the heart is slow to pick up after the contraction is over.

2. *Meconium staining of the liquor.* This is said to be due to contraction of the foetal bowel as a result of hypoxia. The greater the amount of staining the more severe the hypoxia. Staining may be recognized before rupture of the membranes by amnioscopy.

3. *Tumultuous foetal movement*, which is a late sign of hypoxia and may immediately precede death.

These classical signs have long been recognized and have been of great value as a warning that the foetus is in jeopardy, but sometimes sudden foetal death may occur without warning and further methods of recognizing danger have recently been developed. Of these perhaps the most widely used are foetal monitoring by cardiotocograph and scalp blood sampling. A variety of instruments has been devised for the former purpose, but all of them provide by electronic means a graphic record of foetal heart rate together with an indication of the strength of uterine contractions and the relation of the two. Several studies have clearly shown the many deficiencies and inaccuracies of clinical methods of auscultation of the foetal heart, and it is hoped that the improved accuracy of the electronic observations may give earlier warning of the foetus at risk and so improve salvage. Foetal scalp blood sampling is dependent upon the fact that oxygen deprivation leads to increasing acidosis of the foetus, and that this is reflected in the pH of his blood; the lower the figure the greater the acidity and the greater the risk to the foetus. With the aid of an amnioscope, a minute incision is made in the foetal scalp with a special knife and a capillary tube applied, whereby a sample of blood may be assessed in a pH meter. If the figure falls below 7·25, the foetus is in imminent danger and termination of pregnancy is urgently required.

16

Intervention in labour

Where the mother is unable by her own efforts to deliver her baby in good condition or where labour is so prolonged as to endanger mother or child, intervention is called for. Whether this should aim at assisted vaginal delivery or whether abdominal delivery is called for will depend upon the circumstances of each individual case.

Indications for intervention have been considered in Chapter 15, but this may be required also in prolapsed cord (Chapter 19), abnormal presentations and lies (Chapter 10), toxaemia (Chapter 13), heart or lung disease (Chapter 20) and many other conditions.

Where labour ceases to progress or where maternal or foetal conditions demand delivery, one must consider whether vaginal delivery would pe practicable and whether it would offer the best solution to the problem presented. If not abdominal delivery must be undertaken by *Caesarean section*. This operation, reputedly named after Julius Caesar, who it seems was *not* delivered abdominally, is of great antiquity and was practised in Ancient Egypt, usually after the death of the mother. Through the ages it seems to have been practised, but it was only towards the end of the 19th century, with all the technical improvements in abdominal surgery, that the results justified its use. Since then, with improvements not only in technique and in anaesthesia but also in the nutrition of the patient, the avoidance of anaemia and the greater availability of blood transfusion and the better control of infection, Caesarean section has become much less hazardous than a difficult vaginal delivery, and consequently much more commonly employed than in the past. In many units dealing with complicated obstetrics the incidence of Caesarean section may reach 10 per cent or more. Furthermore, one of the objections to Caesarean section, that it tended to limit family size, has lost much of its validity, since attitudes have turned against large families and excessive increase in population. A difficult vaginal delivery may well leave a permanently damaged mother and a defective baby, and so Caesarean section is usually to be preferred. On the other hand, when it is considered that vaginal delivery will be safe for mother and baby, this should be the method of choice.

CAESAREAN SECTION

The classical operation in which the child was delivered through a vertical incision near the fundus has been replaced almost completely by the lower segment operation which uses a low transverse incision, which is less likely to rupture in a future pregnancy and, if it does, will be complicated by much less bleeding, with lower risk to mother and baby. There is less risk of adhesions between the uterine scar and the small bowel, and so the risk of future intestinal obstruction is less. It is very rarely that the classical operation is to be preferred, but where access to the lower segment would be very difficult, as for example in severe kyphosis, it may be the operation of choice.

In the lower segment operation, the utero-vesical peritoneum is cut across, the lower segment exposed and a transverse incision made wide enough to facilitate extraction of the infant. As this is carried out, Ergometrine 0·5 mg is injected intravenously by the anaesthetist, and the placenta and membranes removed. Accurate coaptation of the edges of the uterine wound is of great importance, and sutures should be placed through the whole thickness of the muscle but excluding the decidua, to avoid a weak scar. Sterilization may be carried out if required before closure of the abdominal wall.

Following Caesarean section in one pregnancy, the operation should be repeated in future pregnancies if the same indication persists. If however the indication for the first section is non-recurrent then it may be proper to seek vaginal delivery in the future, and in many cases labour after previous section may be rapidly and easily completed. If not, forceps or ventouse application may be advisable to reduce the strain on the scar. In any event, each successive vaginal delivery should be regarded as imposing an added strain on the scar, and after two or more such deliveries it may be prudent to consider sterilization (Chapter 21). In some cases labour is unsatisfactory and it may be decided, after a suitable trial, that repeat section will be required. In all cases where a repeat section is decided upon, it may be found that the scar is so weak and thin that a further pregnancy would carry a severe risk of uterine rupture. In these cases the surgeon is well advised to obtain from the patient and her husband authority to sterilize her if he considers it essential. In the case of a third section most surgeons advise routine sterilization since the technical difficulty and complications increase with each successive operation, and with them the risks to the mother.

THE OBSTETRIC FORCEPS

Hundreds of obstetric forceps of different patterns have been devised over the past 350 years and a number of different types are in use today. The usual design includes a pair of blades curved in two directions, firstly a cephalic curve designed to fit the head of the infant and secondly a pelvic curve which is intended to match the curve of the pelvis. At their distal ends the blades are linked by a cross-over lock, and then pass on to form handles of various sizes and

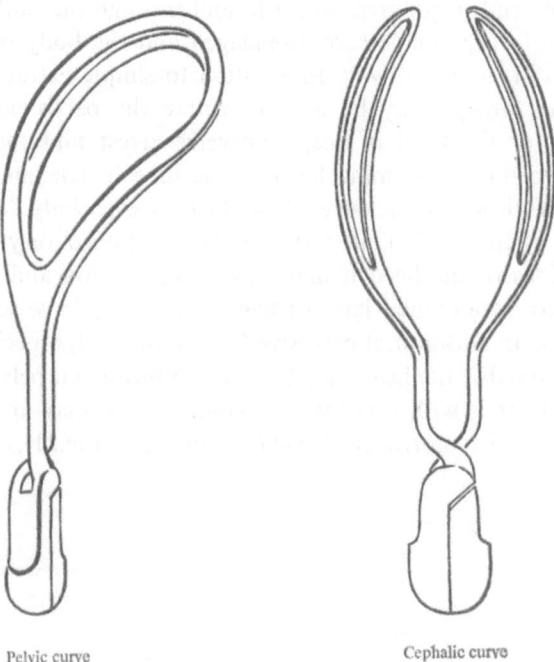

Pelvic curve   Cephalic curve

Fig.31. Wrigley's forceps.

shapes. The blades are inserted separately to lie on either side of the head and then locked together so that the handles are opposed and the blades encircle and grasp the head. In the latter years of the nineteenth and the early years of the present century various traction rods and other devices were designed so as to permit axis traction, i.e. to enable the operator to draw the head down in the axis of the pelvis even when it still lay at a high level; direct traction on the handles in these cases would merely pull the head against the pubis, and seriously militate against successful delivery. The importance of the axis traction principle has greatly diminished in recent years, since the more heroic type of vaginal delivery has given way to freer use of Caesarean section; high forceps delivery, i.e. delivery initiated when the head still remains above mid-cavity or even above the brim, has been shown to be so dangerous for both mother and child that it has been almost completely abandoned except occasionally in the case of a second twin. Mid-cavity forceps are applied to the head which has reached the level of the ischial spines and low forceps when the head has reached the perineum. Traction applied to the handles (or the axis traction handles) will assist the head to progress down to and through the outlet. At this point the forceps blades are disengaged and the body of the child delivered in the usual way. In addition to simple extraction of the head, the forceps may be used to rotate the persistent occipito-posterior or the head in deep transverse arrest and may also be applied to the aftercoming head of the breech. Kielland's forceps (Fig.32) with less pelvic curve than most are especially designed for rotation of the head. Unless the forceps is applied very accurately to the sides of the head it may cause compression and distortion, leading to intra-cranial haemorrhage which may have serious consequences. In addition, if excessive force is applied, especially in the premature baby, the head may be dragged through a pelvis which is too small for it with excessive moulding, which may also result in intra-cranial haemorrhage. Wrigley's forceps (Fig.31), which are

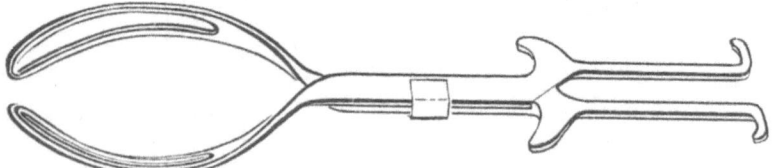

Fig.32. Kielland's forceps.

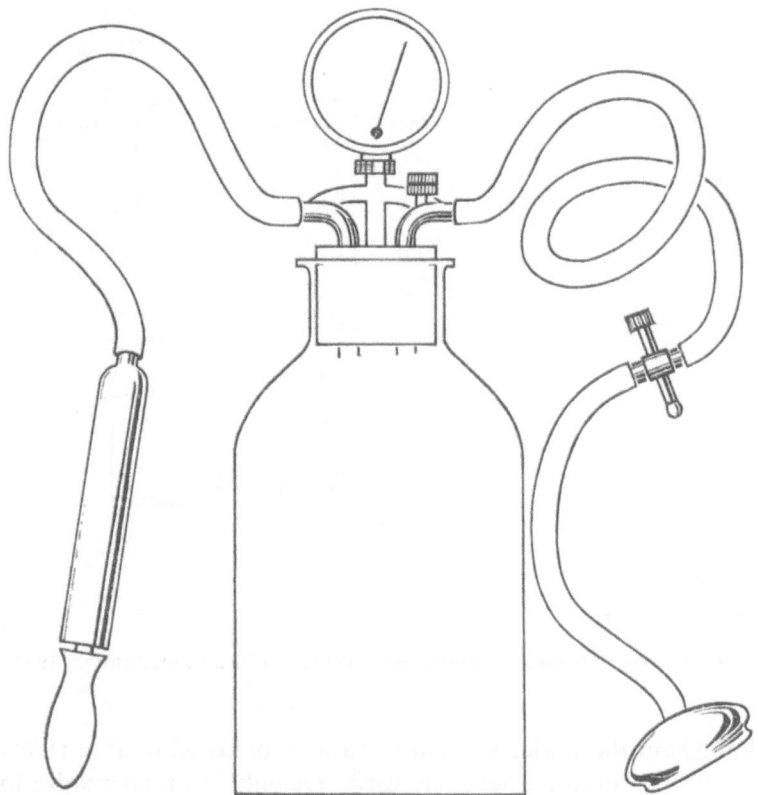

Fig.33. The Malmström vacuum extractor or ventouse (1957).

widely used for low 'lift-out' deliveries, are of light construction with small handles which make the use of excessive force virtually imposs ible.

The forceps should not be applied before full dilatation of the cervix, and are dangerous if the head lies above the level of the spines. They may often be useful in mid-cavity arrest of the head, and the low operation, especially with Wrigley's forceps, may safely lead to considerable shortening of the second stage of labour.

THE VENTOUSE

The application of a vacuum cup to the head of the foetus to assist delivery was first suggested in 1704 but although many different instruments were devised during the next 250 years, the Malmström vacuum extractor (Fig.33) of 1957 was the first to receive wide acceptance

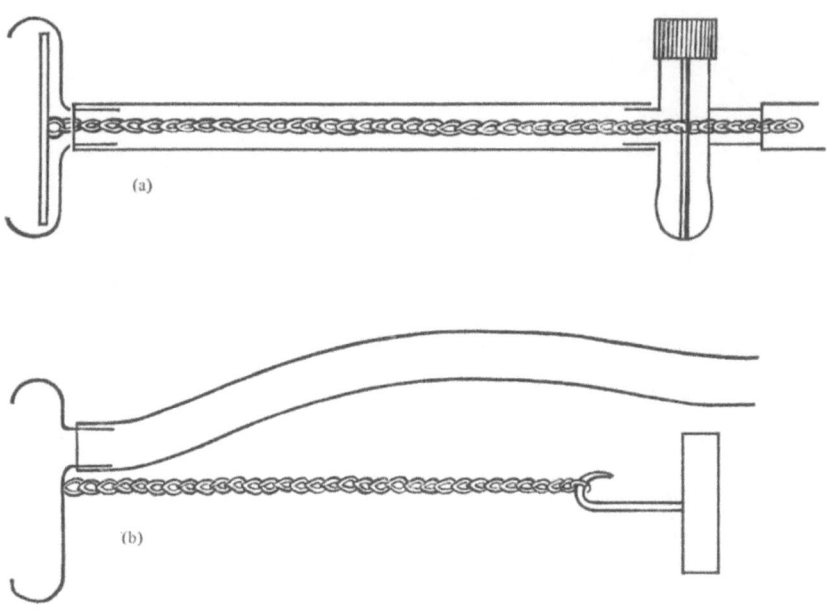

Fig.34. The vacuum cup, (*a.*) Malmström, 1957; (*b.*) Bird's modification, 1968

throughout the world. It has been further improved by Bird (1968)
and in this form is extensively used, not only as an alternative to
forceps but also to deal with situations for which the forceps is
unsuitable (Fig.34). The ventouse, as the instrument is commonly
called in this country, consists of a range of metal cups, 40, 50 and
60 mm in diameter with incurved edges, linked to a traction handle and
to a vacuum system whereby the air from the cup can be exhausted.
A hand-pump or a more elaborate electric pump may be used for this
purpose. A cup of appropriate size is selected and applied to the head
of the child, and a vacuum induced by stages until a negative pressure
of $-0\cdot8$ Kg per cm^2 is reached. This causes the development of an
artificial caput succedaneum or chignon, which fills the cup so that
considerable traction force may be applied without detachment.
As a result the head may be drawn down the birth canal and delivered
with much less risk of compression than with the forceps. The
ventouse may be applied using one of the smaller cups before full
dilatation of the cervix and will usually effect dilatation and delivery
surprisingly rapidly. Dilatation is probably effected by the pressure
of the head drawn down with the ventouse on to the upper aspect

of the cervix, and so stimulating improved activity of the upper uterine segment. In addition if the cup is applied well back towards the occiput, it will effect flexion of the persistent occipito-posterior or deep transversely arrested head so as to promote rotation in a much more physiological way than is possible with forceps or even manually. Rotation, especially in an anthropoid pelvis, will often be posterior with subsequent face to pubis delivery. The ventouse imposes no constraint upon the head as regards level, direction, rate and speed of rotation in contrast to the completely artificial situation with the forceps. The chignon is a formidable swelling, but it rapidly abates, and although some scalp trauma may occur it is seldom serious. Several comparative studies have shown in general that the results of ventouse delivery are significantly better for mother and child than those of the forceps.

EPISIOTOMY AND PERINEAL LACERATION

In a very large proportion of primigravid and in some multiparous labours, tearing will occur as the perineum is stretched by the emerging foetal head, leading to perineal laceration of greater or less extent. Tearing of the introital skin fold (fourchette) is almost invariable and is described as first degree laceration. Second degree tears extend back as far as or alongside the anal margin, whilst if the anal sphincter is involved the tear is classed as third degree. *Episiotomy* is an incision deliberately made into the perineum, generally with scissors to prevent irregular laceration or to limit its extent. In addition it may be used where the advance of the head is held up on the perineum, especially with a premature infant, where it may obviate the use of the forceps or ventouse, and to improve access to the birth canal when manipulations such as forceps, ventouse or breech delivery are undertaken. The posterior end of the labium majus is occupied by a large plexus of veins; in order to avoid damage to this, episiotomy should always begin in the mid-line and be angled so as to avoid the anal sphincter.

The repair of episiotomy or of lacerations should be carried out as soon as possible after delivery, but in the case of a third degree tear, this should be performed under general anaesthesia with full theatre facilities to try to ensure accurate repair of the sphincter. As a rule, the vaginal wounds are first closed, then the levators brought across and the perineal body re-constituted, and finally the perineal skin closed. A third degree tear is almost always associated with tearing of the anterior rectal wall, and is easily recognized by the exposure of the smooth pink posterior rectal wall. In this case, the anterior rectal wall is closed and the torn ends of the sphincter recovered and sutured. Thereafter, the repair is completed as for a second degree tear. In the puerperium, laxatives such as psyllium (Isogel) are of value in ensuring softening of the stool; if these are used there is no need to inhibit bowel movement, which in any case is likely to be delayed until about the third day.

ANAESTHESIA IN OBSTETRICS

Obstetric anaesthesia may constitute one of the most difficult problems which the anaesthetist has to face, and the increasing share of total maternal mortality which is attributed to anaesthesia confirms this. The danger lies principally in Mendleson's syndrome. During labour gastric emptying is delayed and a highly acid semifluid content accumulates in the stomach. During the induction of general anaesthesia, regurgitation and inhalation of this highly acid material may be followed by severe shock and bronchospasm, leading to extreme collapse and sometimes death. This led for some years to the avoidance of general anaesthesia. Instead, local and spinal anaesthesia was used for Caesarean section but the former was quite often inadequate and the latter lethal. The heavy uterus of late pregnancy pressing upon the inferior vena cava as the patient lies on her back leads to interruption of the venous return to the heart, hypotension and fainting (supine hypotensive syndrome). When the hypotension so often associated with spinal anaesthesia is superadded to this, fatal collapse may occur. Treatment by rolling the patient on her side should be rapidly effective and may be lifesaving. The present practice in Caesarean section is to avoid food (even fluids) by mouth for 4 hours at least before operation, to empty the stomach by means of a Ryle's tube which remains in situ throughout operation, and to place magnesium trisilicate or some other antacid in the stomach prior to operation. Anaesthesia is induced with the patient's head high and a cuffed endotracheal tube introduced as promptly as possible. Although 'smash and grab' techniques have been condemned, it has recently been shown that the oxygen tension in the cord blood of the infant delivered after some delay is significantly lower than that of the infant delivered promptly after induction of anaesthesia. For this reason the opening of the uterus and extraction of the infant should be accomplished as promptly as possible so as to spare him this effect of anaesthesia.

For vaginal delivery, local infiltration of the perineum is commonly used as a preliminary to episiotomy, using ½–1 per cent lignocaine. For assisted deliveries *pudendal nerve-block* regional anaesthesia may be achieved by supplementing this perineal infiltration with 10 ml of ½–1 per cent lignocaine placed in the region of the ischial spine on either side. Care must be taken to avoid intravenous injection which may cause collapse. *Paracervical block* using marcaine has been used for some years but, although many good results have been reported, a number of poorly explained infant deaths has occurred and so the method has not become widely popular. *Epidural block* can provide good and long-lasting anaesthesia, but this too may be associated with collapse and also post-delivery headaches and pareses, and so is best undertaken by skilled anaesthetists. Once the uterus is empty, general anaesthesia for example in retained placenta seems to be less hazardous, but still carries certain risks. It is clear therefore that obstetric anaesthesia should not be undertaken by the unskilled and there is a strong move afoot for the provision of full-time cover by consultant anaesthetists in every obstetric unit.

17

The Rhesus factor

The Rhesus factor (Rh) is an antigen capable of stimulating the production of antibodies if introduced into an individual whose organism does not normally contain it. It is present as a normal constituent in the blood and other cells of about 80 per cent of Europeans, who are described as Rhesus positive. In the remaining 20 per cent it is absent, and these individuals are Rhesus negative. The Rhesus status is independent of the ABO groups.

The Rhesus factor may be introduced into the Rh negative individual in several ways. A transfusion of Rhesus positive blood into a Rhesus negative patient will be strongly antigenic and produce antibodies in high titre. Similarly, intramuscular injection of blood of another individual, which used to be carried out in certain dermatological clinics especially for allergic eczema in children, may still bring sensitized individuals to the obstetrician. A bizarre case was reported from a well-known boarding school for girls on the South Coast where two little girls, one Rhesus positive and the second Rhesus negative, decided in token of their eternal friendship to mix their blood obtained from small incisions in their forearms. The Rhesus negative girl was sensitized, as was discovered many years later when she became pregnant. The most common way in which the Rh antigen may be introduced into the body of a Rhesus negative individual is when a Rhesus negative mother has a Rhesus positive husband, and conceives a Rhesus positive child. Unless she is previously sensitized, her first pregnancy will almost certainly be unaffected clinically. The actual sensitization almost always occurs as the result of foeto-maternal transfusion from the placenta, either during the separation in the third stage of labour or as a result of earlier separation associated with ante-partum haemorrhage or occasionally with abortion. Foetal cells may thus enter the mother's blood stream, and this rapidly gives rise to the formation of anti-bodies.

The Rhesus factor is inherited through a dominant gene from one or both of one's parents or from neither. If it is inherited from both parents the offspring is said to be homozygous Rhesus positive. If it is inherited from only one parent the offspring will be hetero-zygous Rhesus positive. Only when it is inherited from neither parent will the offspring be Rhesus negative. In this way, two heterozygous parents may have either a Rh negative or a Rh positive child. The Rh factor has at least three possible antigens C, D, and E, of which the D is clinically the most important. By testing the individual against specific test sera, his genotype, i.e. his status in relation to all these antigens, may be determined and expressed with a double triad of letters, large or small. Rh positivity is expressed in capital and negativity in small letters. Thus a genotype CDe/cDe with capitals on both sides indicates a homozygous Rh positive, cDe/cde is heterozygous Rhesus positive. The genotype of a Rh negative indi-vidual is expressed as cde/cde.

The clinical importance of the Rh factor in obstetrics is the possible occurrence of haemolytic disease of the newborn child of a Rh negative woman. If the woman is Rh positive, the antigen is a normal constituent of her body and will not stimulate the formation of antibodies even if introduced from another individual. The child of a first pregnancy of a Rh negative mother with a Rh positive husband will almost invariably escape as we have seen, but in subsequent pregnancies, antibodies may build up in the mother's blood stream, cross the placenta to the blood stream of the infant and attack his red cells so as to cause haemolysis. Red cells become swollen and rupture, so that their haemoglobin enters the serum where it is converted to bilirubin. Not only does this lead to anaemia, but if the serum bilirubin accumulates in the blood to a level above 20–25 mg per cent the infant is in danger of kernicterus or jaundice of the basal nuclei of the brain. This destroys the cells of these nuclei to such an extent that the infant may die or survive with severe and irreversible mental and physical handicap. In the premature infant, whose liver is immature and unable adequately to destroy the excess bilirubin, an even lower figure than I have quoted may be associated with harmful effects.

HYDROPS FOETALIS

If the husband of a Rh negative woman is heterozygous, half of his sperms will carry the gene for the Rh factor, and half will not do so. Half of his children therefore may be expected to be Rh positive and half Rh negative. The Rh negative children, like the first Rh positive child, will be unaffected, but all subsequent Rh positive children are likely to be more and more severely affected until the stage of hydrops foetalis is reached. This is a condition of general anasarca with ascites and pleural and pericardial effusion, which is incompatible with survival. It may be diagnosed in utero by the large size of the foetus, and by the fact that X-ray may show that he adopts the Buddha position with his legs splayed out on either side of his swollen belly, and that there is a halo of oedematous soft tissues around the bony outline of the skull.

The condition should be easily diagnosed and all pregnant women should be tested for antibody formation. (ABO antibodies may often be found, and although they are rarely of clinical importance, they may produce effects similar to those of the Rhesus factor.) A rising titre of antibodies will indicate that the foetus is likely to be severely affected as will a history of previously affected children. The affected child will be jaundiced at birth or at latest within 24 hours, and cord-blood haemoglobin and serum bilirubin will be found to be lowered and raised respectively. (The normal haemoglobin level of the new-born is about 130 per cent, so that a figure of 80 per cent or less represents a severe anaemia.)

In addition the blood of the child should be grouped, and his Rhesus status determined. If he is ABO compatible, the risk of severe affection is greater; ABO incompatibility on the other hand is to some extent protective. If the child is Rhesus negative, he will not be affected and some other cause of any anaemia and jaundice must be sought.

The Coombs test should always be carried out on the cord blood at birth. If positive it indicates that sensitization has occurred. If it is negative, Rh sensitization can be excluded.

Amniocentesis may have a role from quite early in pregnancy. If the titre of antibodies is high or rising steeply, a specimen of liquor amnii may be obtained by transabdominal puncture after the 24th week and its optical density at 450 Ångstrom units recorded and compared with the normal range from charts prepared by Liley.

Care must be taken to avoid puncture of the placenta by accurate localization as described in Chapter 11. Puncture of the placenta may lead to further foeto-maternal transfusion or to retro-placental haemorrhage, and to contamination of the liquor which will vitiate not only the current results but also those of future amniocentesis.

Amnioscopy in which the forewaters are inspected by means of a telescope passed through the cervical canal may also be helpful in diagnosis by revealing yellow discolouration of the liquor.

TREATMENT

Treatment may be entirely conservative. The mother in whom antibodies are found should always be confined in a department where the child can be accurately monitored. The cord blood findings at birth should be considered and if the haemoglobin level is above 80 per cent and the serum bilirubin no more than 5·0 mg per cent, most paediatricians will be prepared to await events and to see what the figures will be like after 6–12 hours. If the cord-blood findings are less satisfactory, or if the later tests show marked deterioration and in particular if the serum bilirubin concentration rises rapidly towards a figure that threatens kernicterus, active treatment is indicated. On the other hand, with relatively satisfactory cord-blood findings and slow initial deterioration, it may be justifiable to continue to await events. Haemoglobin and serum bilirubin must be checked daily or more often and in many cases will reach a peak about the fifth day of life and fall away thereafter as the antibodies are eliminated from the body of the child.

In the more severely affected cases one or more exchange transfusions with ABO compatible Rh negative blood, which will not be attacked by the anti-Rh antibodies, will be required. Through a polythene catheter introduced into the umbilical vein 10 ml of child's blood is withdrawn and replaced with 10 ml of donor blood. This is repeated until about 20–25 ml per pound body weight have been exchanged. By this time, about 75–80 per cent of the circulating cells should be Rh negative, and so likely to survive until the antibodies have finally been eliminated. In the worst cases, a further climb in serum bilirubin figures may indicate repeat transfusion once or even more often. Most of the antibodies will have been destroyed by the 10th–14th day, and if kernicterus has been avoided up to this stage there is likely to be no further trouble.

In order to offer hope of salvage of the worst affected children, who would suffer hydrops and either die in utero or very soon after birth, the technique of intra-uterine transfusion of Rh negative blood has been developed during the past decade. Through a long needle passed through the abdominal and uterine walls of the mother and the abdominal wall of the foetus, about 20 ml Rh negative blood is placed in the peritoneal cavity of the child and this may be repeated every 10–14 days. By means of this technique the child is kept alive in utero, and it is claimed that hydrops may be reversed. Induction of labour is performed at about 35 weeks and exchange transfusion carried out as described above. By this means, many children have survived whose elder siblings had died in utero or soon after birth. Even where intra-uterine transfusion is not considered to be necessary, induction of labour may be indicated in cases where a previous child has died in the last weeks of pregnancy, and the obstetric history of each case must be carefully studied with this possibility in mind.

PREVENTION OF Rh SENSITIZATION

Prevention of Rh sensitization has recently become possible, since the importance of foeto-maternal transfusion at the time of delivery has been recognized. The presence of foetal cells in the blood of the newly-delivered mother can be recognized by the Kleihauer-Betke technique where a stained blood film is treated with acid. This leads to fading of the colouration of adult red cells, but foetal haemo-globin resists this, and the well-stained foetal cells will stand out in the film. If anti-D gamma-globulin is given to the mother within 72 hours of delivery, the formation of antibodies will be prevented, so that her next child will be free from the risk of Rh haemolytic disease. At first, supplies of the gamma-globulin were obtained only from mothers sensitized to the D factor, and treatment was restricted to mother's showing foetal red cells after delivery. Today, more adequate supplies of gamma-globulin are being obtained following the sensitization of Rh negative male volunteers, and it is advocated that all Rh negative mothers having a Rh positive child should be treated in this way. As a result of the comprehensive prophylactic treatment of all mothers whose future children are at risk, it is to be hoped that Rh haemolytic disease will cease to be a problem. It should be stressed however that where antibodies are already present, this method has nothing to offer; it is important therefore that every Rh negative mother of a Rh positive child be treated promptly after her first delivery, and also after every subsequent delivery of a Rh positive child.

18

Venereal diseases in pregnancy

Venereal diseases by definition are infections usually affecting the genital organs transmitted by sexual intercourse. The various organisms concerned are incapable of survival outside the body, and direct bodily contact is necessary for their transmission. In recent years there has been a steady increase in incidence of both syphilis and gonorrhoea, the two most important venereal diseases of this country. Lymphogranuloma venereum is found as a venereal disease in the tropics but is rare in this country. Chancroid and soft chancre are occasionally found in Mediterranean countries but rarely present in Britain. Vaginitis due to trichomonas vaginalis or to candida albicans (thrush) may be sexually transmitted. They may co-exist with each other, with gonorrhoea and with syphilis, and so a diagnosis of trichomoniasis or candidiasis must not lead one to over-look the possibility of a more serious infection.

GONORRHOEA

Gonorrhoea may arise during pregnancy or before it. It is due to the gonococcus, a Gram negative diplococcus, which may be grown from gonorrhoeal discharges. The disease in the female commonly presents as an acute inflammation involving urethra, cervix, Bartholin's and Skene's (urethral) glands, with profuse purulent discharge from these various sites arising 2–3 days after the infecting intercourse. It will usually respond promptly to one or two mega-units of penicillin, but many resistant strains have been described, and in such cases, or in the untreated case, the infection may involve the upper genital tract, giving rise to an acute salpingitis. This may later become chronic and cause infertility due to tubal obstruction and to chronic pelvic inflammatory disease. Rarely the condition may cause peritonitis, pericarditis or arthritis, and involvement of the eyes may cause blindness.

Treatment should usually be undertaken by the venereology department, since the organization for tests of cure as well as contact tracing is usually better there than in the ante-natal clinic, but the patient should be referred as promptly as possible to try to ensure that she is free from infection by the time she goes into labour.

In obstetrics we are particularly concerned with the effect that an inadequately treated infection may have upon the child, even years after the acute infection has subsided. In such a case, the organism may persist in the fastnesses of the cervical glands, whence it may be expressed during labour when the head of the child passes through the birth canal. As a result, ophthalmia neonatorum may ensue. This will present as a furious pan-ophthalmitis usually within 24 hours of birth, with very profuse creamy purulent discharge and such marked oedema of the eyelids that it may be difficult to see the acutely inflamed cornea. Blindness may well result if active treatment is not instituted promptly, and as soon as swabs have been obtained for bacteriological examination penicillin should be administered both systematically and as eye drops. These cases can usually be distinguished from the much more common 'sticky eye' on clinical grounds alone because of their extreme severity and usually earlier onset. The advice of an ophthalmic surgeon may be desirable.

SYPHILIS

Syphilis is a disease of great antiquity due to a treponemal organism called the Spirochaete pallida. The primary manifestation is usually an ulcerated lesion most commonly on the genital tract, called a chancre, with associated swelling and tenderness of regional lymph glands, and this appears some 10–21 days after the infecting intercourse. The spirochaete may be demonstrated by dark ground illumination in scrapings from the ulcer. If untreated, it may regress only to be followed after 6–12 weeks by generalized secondary syphilis, with rashes, pyrexia and general malaise. Tertiary and post-tertiary syphilis may occur many years later and almost any organ of the body may be affected, and heart disease, strokes, paralysis, blindness, deafness and dementia may result. If treatment is instituted promptly on the appearance of the primary lesion, the disease may often be cured with penicillin one mega-unit daily for 15 days, but here also resistant organisms have been reported, and, as with gonorrhoea, treatment is best carried out in the venereology department. The serological tests for syphilis such as the Wassermann and Kahn reactions do not become positive until some weeks after the appearance of the primary lesion, but then they may remain positive for life.

Here again, the obstetrician is particularly concerned with the risk that a mother may transmit the disease to her baby, who may be aborted (usually in the second trimester) or stillborn. Even if the child survives as a congenital syphilitic, he will be subject to all the disastrous disabilities of the late stages of syphilis, but at an early age. Suggestive signs in the newborn are rhagades (fissuring at the angles of the mouth), snuffles (purulent nasal discharge), the 'syphilitic wig' (the hair is patchy and unhealthy-looking with areas of baldness) and later Hutchinson's teeth (notched upper incisors). Later again, interstitial keratitis may cause blindness and juvenile general paralysis of the insane may produce progressive dementia and death. It is clearly incumbent upon all those responsible for the care of the pregnant woman to leave no stone unturned to prevent this appalling situation, and so it is generally recommended that every woman have a Wassermann reaction in every pregnancy with such confirmatory tests as are considered necessary. Occasional false positive tests are found; if a positive result does occur, it should be repeated and other tests added. Should these again be positive, the patient should be referred to the venereologist for treatment as soon as possible. If treatment, usually with penicillin, can be completed some weeks before term, one should be confident of obtaining a healthy child. It is a wise precaution however to obtain a cord-blood Wassermann reaction and to treat the neonate if any doubt exists.

TRICHOMONIASIS

Trichomoniasis rarely seems to affect the infant but the mother (and probably the father also) should be treated with metronidazole once the period of organogenesis is past.

CANDIDIASIS

Candidiasis of the maternal vagina may be transmitted to the infant to cause oral thrush. This may cause much soreness and give rise to feeding difficulties, and it may spread to the lungs to cause a dangerous fungal pneumonia. For this reason, active treatment with nystatin or other fungicides should be undertaken as soon as infection is recognized during pregnancy.

19

The foetus and his environment

Whilst the study of the newborn is more properly the field of the paediatrician, the obstetrician must concern himself with many aspects of pregnancy which may affect foetal well-being, and some of these will be discussed in this chapter.

THE PLACENTA

The placenta, as we have seen in Chapter 3, is developed as an aggregation of chorionic villi, and about the twelfth week of pregnancy takes on a variety of functions.

Respiratory function. It is the respiratory mechanism of the foetus, and effects the transfer of oxygen from the mother's blood to that of the foetus and of carbon dioxide in the reverse direction.

Endocrine function. Its endocrine function, which it takes over from the corpus luteum about the twelfth week, includes the production of chorionic gonadotrophins, oestrogen and progesterone, relaxin and other hormones.

Nutritive function. Its nutritive activity involves the carry over of amino acids, sugars, and fatty acids to the foetus, as well as vitamins and minerals such as iron, calcium, magnesium and copper required for the building up of the foetal organs.

Barrier function. A barrier function prevents many organisms from reaching the foetus, but there are exceptions, such as those of syphilis and virus of rubella. Antibodies too may pass the placenta, as in the case of anti-Rhesus antibodies.

Excretory function. The foetus also relies largely on the excretory function of the placenta, some urea and other components of foetal urine being transmitted to the maternal blood stream to be excreted finally by the kidneys of the mother.

Anchoring function. Finally the placenta has an anchoring function; in some pregnancies this appears to be defective and this may lead to abortion or later to premature separation of the placenta.

From what we have already learned of the foetus and his environment, it will be clear that the obstetrician has a variety of opportunities to protect the health of the infant. In practice, the paediatrician is presented with sick infants who fall into four main categories; those born prematurely, those born small-for-dates (light-for-dates, dysmature), those sustaining injury during the birth process, and those congenitally malformed. In any particular case, the infant may present features of two or more of these groups, but for convenience they will be considered separately.

THE PREMATURE BABY

An international convention established many years ago still defines a premature infant as one whose birth weight is 2,500G or less. However, we have seen that low birth weight may result from intra-uterine malnutrition resulting from placental insufficiency. Thus the premature infant should be thought of as one *weighing less than 2,500G* at birth *before the 37th week of pregnancy*, but *whose size is appropriate to the gestational age.*

Premature delivery may be associated with multiple pregnancy and hydramnios, and resting patients with these conditions during the latter part of their pregnancies may help to prevent the premature onset of labour. However, the cause of premature labour in the majority of cases is unclear, and although it is recognized to be more common in certain groups of women (e.g. those from the lower social classes and the unmarried) and also in certain individual women, (who appear to have a constitutional tendency to go into labour prematurely), our management will remain unsatisfactory and these babies will continue to occupy much of the time and effort of our paediatric colleagues.

A last group of infants born prematurely are those born following planned premature delivery for reasons either of maternal health (e.g. severe toxaemia) or foetal health (e.g. in diabetic or Rhesus sensitized pregnancy) or the health of both mother and foetus (e.g. severe accidental haemorrhage).

Premature babies are at risk from two main conditions.

1. *Respiratory distress syndrome.* Firstly, soon after birth they may develop respiratory distress syndrome. This results from a lack of a substance in the lungs of the foetus called surfactant which, when present, facilitates the full expansion and maintenance of the lung alveoli. In its absence, the alveoli remain in a collapsed state, and satisfactory respiration is impossible. If the infant can be protected from severe hypoxia and acidosis by adequate oxygenation and the controlled administration of sodium bicarbonate, time will eventually cure the basic defect. However, the above conditions are often difficult to fulfil and the condition is a major cause of neonatal death.

2. *Blood coagulation disorders.* The second condition is a defect in the blood coagulation of the premature infant. This may result in widespread haemorrhages, but those involving the brain, lungs or gastro-intestinal tract pose the most dangerous threat to the newborn infant and may prove fatal.

In addition to these two major causes of death, the relative immaturity of all systems of the premature infant result in such difficulties as apnoeic attacks, poor temperature control, feeding difficulties and inefficient bilirubin metabolism. All of these make the care of the premature infant a highly specialized and exacting task.

THE SMALL-FOR-DATES (LIGHT-FOR-DATES, DYSMATURE) BABY

These infants, which result from a pregnancy in which there has been defective intra-uterine growth of the foetus, are small like the premature infants, but present slightly different problems to the paediatrician. However the obstetrician and midwife are able to improve the outlook for many of these babies by careful ante-natal care.

Mothers who smoke cigarettes are more likely to give birth to a small-for-dates infant, and this provides us with an approach to the prevention of some of these cases. However, in view of the close association of the condition with toxaemia, the management of most cases depends on an early recognition of that condition in the ante-natal clinics. Failure to gain weight during the pregnancy, or slowing of uterine enlargement may be other indications to investigate further the intra-uterine growth and health of the foetus. This may be monitored by serial measurements of urinary oestriol, human placental lactogen, or in some centres by ultrasonic measurement of the growth of the head of the foetus.

If these investigations show that the foetus is increasingly at risk of hypoxia and malnutrition while remaining in utero, then it may be decided to deliver the baby before term, rather than wait for the spontaneous onset of labour. In this case it is clearly important to confirm that the small foetus is truly 'small-for-dates' and not in fact premature due to an inaccurate estimate of the length of gestation. The maturity of the foetus may be estimated by radiology either by the appearance of the femoral and tibial epiphyses around the knee, which should occur after thirty-six weeks, or by measurement of the length of the shaft of the femur, a method recently introduced which should prove more accurate. Liquor amnii, obtained by amniocentesis, and stained with Nile Blue sulphate, should indicate by the proportion of orange-staining fat-containing cells the duration of the pregnancy. By consideration of all the above, one should be able to decide whether the child should be delivered or not, and continued observation will indicate the best time for this.

The small-for-dates infant is first at risk of *birth asphyxia*, and although this problem may beset any infant, it more frequently requires active resuscitative measures in this group of babies (see section on birth asphyxia). Careful monitoring of foetal well-being during labour by serial measurements of foetal heart rate and pattern, foetal electrocardiogram patterns and blood pH values may indicate the need to effect delivery earlier than would be achieved spontaneously. Like the premature infants, these babies also have blood coagulation defects, and may develop fatal haemorrhages into brain, lung or gut.

However, the distinctive problem of this group is *hypoglycaemia* (low blood sugar level) and if this is not actively looked for, the baby may suffer convulsions and brain damage, and possibly die. This is a largely preventable condition and if all small-for-dates infants are recognized before or soon after birth, its virtual elimination should be possible.

THE INFANT INJURED DURING BIRTH

Happily, with the increasingly widespread facilities offered to women delivered in this country, serious injury to the baby at the time of delivery is becoming a rarity. Some groups of infants, such as the premature and small-for-dates babies, are more prone to injury than the fully mature. But even in well-grown babies, a difficult breech or instrumental delivery may be the cause of damage which proves either fatal or to be the cause of persisting disability. The most serious damage sustained in this way is *intra-cranial*. A tear of the falx cerebri (a membranous fold lying vertically between the two cerebral hemispheres), or the tentorium cerebelli (lying above the cerebellum and below the posterior halves of the cerebral hemispheres), results in damage to the venous sinuses (Fig.35) with which they are closely related. The resulting intra-cranial haemorrhage may be immediately fatal, or the infant may die in the neonatal period. The more seriously affected survivors may show subsequent mental or neurological defect (e.g. spastic paralysis).

Other injuries sustained more rarely during difficult or careless delivery may result in *ruptured abdominal viscera* (e.g. spleen or liver), *injured nerves* (e.g. brachial plexus), or *broken bones* (e.g. clavicle, humerus and femur). The conduct of all deliveries in fully-equipped obstetric units will reduce the numbers of babies affected by birth injury still further.

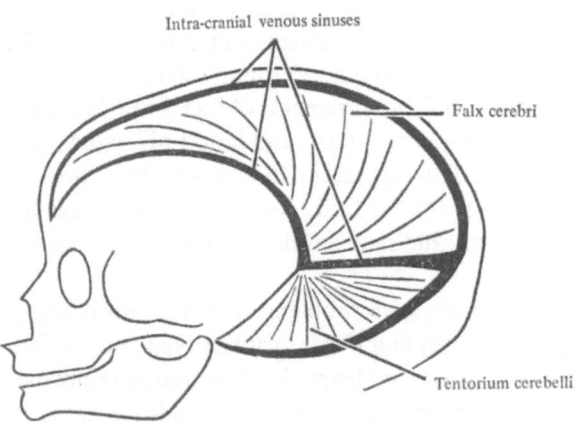

Fig.35. Intra-cranial dural folds and venous sinuses.

THE CONGENITALLY MALFORMED INFANT

A large proportion of abortions are due to abnormalities of embryonic or ovular development; unfortunately not all are eliminated in this way, and many deformed children reach term or nearly so. Some of these suffer abnormalities incompatible with life and are stillborn or die early in the neonatal period, but others survive with various degrees of disability.

Causes

The approach to this problem is difficult because, in general, the cause of the abnormality is not clear. Early pregnancy, when organs are being formed, is a critical period and drugs and viruses have both been shown to have serious effects on the foetus at this stage in its development. Congenital heart disease, blindness, deafness and microcephaly may all result from *rubella* infection, and the tragic appearance of phocomelia following *thalidomide* administration in early pregnancy has led to very careful screening of all drugs given to women.

A better understanding of hereditary disease and the development of genetic counselling services have prompted sterilization in some couples where this is appropriate. It is comparatively rarely, however, that the opportunity to prevent conception of an abnormal foetus presents itself. The discouragement of pregnancy late in life when mongolism is more likely is another example.

In another small group it may be possible to abort the pregnancy if there is a high risk of serious foetal abnormality, and this is so in cases of maternal rubella or exposure to large doses of *ionizing radiation* in early pregnancy. Amniocentesis in early pregnancy may yield helpful information regarding the chromosome pattern of the foetus. For example the early recognition of mongolism (Down's syndrome) in this way might permit termination of the pregnancy. Direct visualization of the foetus with an endoscope inserted into the amniotic sac is in the process of development and may prove a useful additional approach to the recognition of congenital abnormality, early enough to permit termination of pregnancy.

Abnormalities

Anencephaly is commonly associated with hydramnios and in this con-

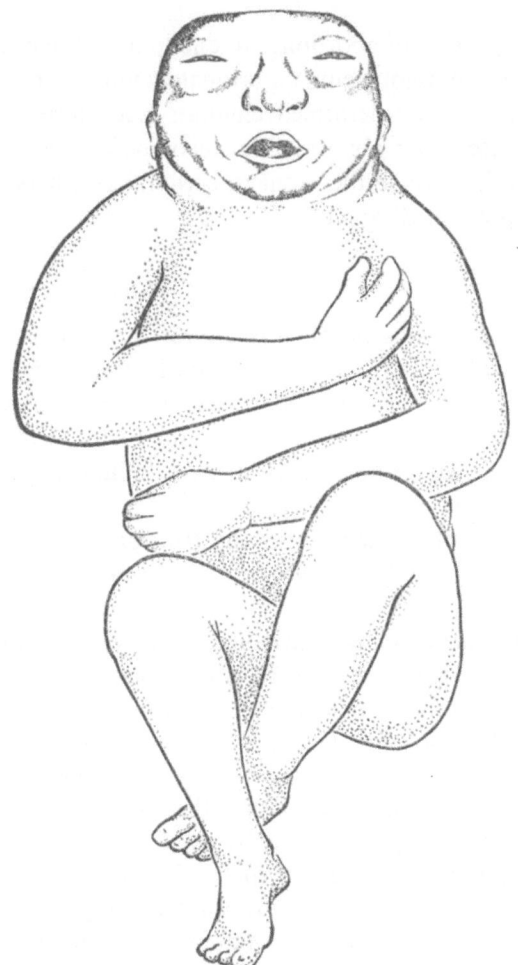

Fig.36. Anencephalic foetus.

dition it is important to X-ray the mother's abdomen in an attempt to demonstrate whether there is any radiological abnormality of the foetus. The anencephalic has a typical X-ray appearance (Fig.36) and diagnosis can be made with certainty. In these cases there is foetal pituitary and adrenal deficiency so that the onset of labour may be delayed, and it is important therefore, to induce labour to rid the mother of her valueless conceptus.

Hydrocephalus should be recognized on clinical grounds by the large compressible head which may lie at the fundus, or by the characteristic feeling of wide sutures ('islands of bone in a sea of membrane') on vaginal examination. The head may be tapped with a spinal needle, or, if the breech presents, through the frequently associated spina bifida, so as to reduce its size sufficiently to enable the head to negotiate the pelvis.

Oesophageal atresia. In hydramnios, if no radiological abnormality of the foetus is demonstrated, there may be an oesophageal atresia, and catheterization of the oesophagus soon after birth with a soft rubber catheter, before any feed is given, is of vital importance.

Geographical and social class differences in the prevalence of some congenital abnormalities is recognized, but the cause of these is not yet clear.

Thus the majority of congenitally abnormal babies continue to be born to apparently normal couples after apparently normal pregnancies, and will only be recognised in the neonatal period or during infancy.

BIRTH ASPHYXIA

The failure of any infant to establish satisfactory respiration at birth may be due to a variety of factors. Predisposing elements in the four groups outlined above may contribute, but an otherwise normal baby may have difficulty in starting to breathe. Cerebral anoxia at this stage of life may be disastrous for future intellectual and neurological development and lead to death of nerve cells which cannot be replaced. Every effort must be made therefore, to maintain oxygenation as early as possible.

Treatment

The condition of the infant is conveniently recorded by means of the *Apgar Score* which awards 2, 1 or 0 points for each of five criteria: respiration, heart beat, muscle tone, reflex activity and skin colour, according to whether these are good, poor or absent. This score should be recorded at 1 and 5 minutes after birth to indicate which resuscitative technique is most appropriate and also to measure its success. The 5 minute score is useful for assessing the prognosis for that particular child.

Aspiration of mucus. The vast majority of babies that fail to breathe satisfactorily at birth will do so after aspiration of mucus, liquor, or meconium blocking the upper airway. This is achieved with a mucus extractor and together with gentle stimulation of the baby either by blowing on the abdomen or lightly flicking the sole of the foot will resolve most cases of transient birth asphyxia.

Aspiration of the larynx. Babies failing to respond to these simple measures require aspiration of the larynx under direct vision with a laryngoscope, followed by the administration of oxygen by intermittent positive pressure ventilation, either with an oro-pharyngeal airway and face mask or, in more severe cases, by endotracheal intubation.

N-allyl normorphine. Occasionally it may be felt that recent sedation of the mother with opiates may be contributing to respiratory depression in the infant in which case n-allyl normorphine may be given, preferably intravenously.

Acidosis and hypoglycaemia may also need correction and in this case sodium bicarbonate and glucose respectively are administered intravenously.

During all resuscitative measures the baby must be kept warm and experienced paediatric assistance should be summoned as early as possible.

SUMMARY

Midwives are in a strong position to contribute to the successful outcome of pregnancies under their care. During pregnancy they can recognize failure to gain weight, failure of uterine growth, and the onset of hypertension and proteinuria; they can discourage mothers from cigarette smoking while pregnant. During labour the observations of the midwife and timely summoning of medical assistance will often make the difference between a stillbirth and the birth of a live, healthy infant. Her employment of simple resuscitative measures to the baby failing to breathe at birth and her early recognition of the small-for-dates baby may radically affect the life potential of the young patient entrusted to her care, and ensure the happy outcome of a pregnancy.

20

Some medical disorders in pregnancy

Many medical diseases and disabilities have an effect upon pregnancy, but only one or two of the most important can be discussed here.

DIABETES MELLITUS

The effect of pregnancy upon pre-existing diabetes is usually to disturb control. Patients previously well-controlled on long-acting insulins may require soluble insulin, and insulin requirements may fluctuate considerably, sometimes in an upward and sometimes in a downward direction. This instability appears by the second month of pregnancy and continues until a week or two after delivery, so that close supervision by the diabetic physician is essential throughout this period.

Effects on pregnancy

The effects of diabetes upon pregnancy are also marked. There is an increased incidence of abortion, foetal deformity, hydramnios, toxaemia and intra-uterine death.

Hydramnios, an excess of liquor amnii over about 2 litres, is often associated with ovular anomalies, especially those involving failure to swallow such as anencephaly and oesophageal atresia. It may occur in twins, especially uni-ovular, and in diabetes even when no foetal anomaly is present.

Toxaemia is common and often severe, leading to extensive placental infarction, but this may be enhanced by vascular damage to the placenta as a result of the diabetes itself.

Intra-uterine death. Probably in consequence of this, intra-uterine death frequently occurs in the last weeks of pregnancy, rates as high as 40 per cent being quoted in the literature. The children of a diabetic tend to be very large, often as much as 5,000G at 36–37 weeks but they behave as prematures despite their huge size. The outlook for the child is materially improved by strict control of blood sugar throughout the pregnancy, and the closest cooperation between obstetrician and diabetic physician is of great importance. It is usual to terminate the pregnancy soon after the end of the 37th week, and Caesarean section is frequently required, both because of the large size of the child and because of the critical inadequacy of the placenta. Serial oestriol estimations may help the choice of the time of intervention.

Diabetes may first manifest itself during pregnancy, and even before this occurs, pregnancy may be complicated in a manner typical of diabetes—the so-called *pre-diabetic state.* In such a case the birth of a large child (over 4,500G) will indicate a glucose tolerance test which may show a diabetic pattern even in the absence of any clinical evidence of the disease.

The children at birth require very careful paediatric care, and are greatly at risk from respiratory distress syndrome and also from hypoglycaemia. Despite their large size, they are particularly susceptible to infection and even if they are born alive, further losses may occur in the neonatal period.

CARDIAC DISEASE IN PREGNANCY

It is usual to regard heart disease in pregnancy, whether it is congenital or acquired, in terms of functional capacity of the heart and the New York Heart Association Classification of 1939 is still widely used, although its value has recently been questioned. Women with heart disease are classified in 4 grades:

I—no limitation of physical activity.

II—slight limitation. Comfortable at rest, but undue fatigue, palpitation, dyspnoea on exertion.

III—comfortable at rest, but slight activity causes fatigue, dyspnoea etc.

IV—Symptoms present even at rest. Any exertion causes severe discomfort.

Soon after the onset of pregnancy the blood volume begins to increase and by the 12th week it has risen by 30 per cent. The pulse rate remains more or less unchanged in the normal woman and so the stroke volume is greatly increased as is work of the heart. This increased burden is already maximal by the 12th week, and changes little for the remainder of pregnancy. As a result, a woman with heart disease may show decompensation from quite an early stage in pregnancy, and here again, the help of the cardiologist must be sought. In a few cases cardiac surgery during pregnancy may be undertaken with benefit.

In general, patients in Grade I and II will go through pregnancy without undue risk, although they should be under the care of the cardiologist so that treatment may be begun at the first sign of decompensation with bed rest and digitalisation. The prognosis is less good in Grade III and prolonged bed rest is likely to be required. The patient in Grade IV who becomes pregnant is in grave danger, and even if abortion is undertaken, once the pregnancy has reached 8–10 weeks interruption does not appear to improve the diagnosis. A patient may be found to deteriorate from one pregnancy to the next, and there is a strong case for sterilisation in these circumstances. Not infrequently acute cardiac failure arises three or four days after delivery and so intervention should be postponed until at least the 10th day.

In the management of labour, adequate sedation is essential, with assisted delivery as soon as the second stage is reached, or even earlier with the ventouse. Caesarean section is advised only for purely obstetric reasons—as far as the heart disease is concerned, the more rapid haemodynamic changes in Caesarean section as compared with vaginal delivery mean that the latter imposes less of a burden upon the diseased heart.

ANAEMIA OF PREGNANCY

This is a common complication of pregnancy and may take several forms. It is of the utmost importance that a good haemoglobin level be maintained in order to promote optimal function of heart, lungs, placenta and kidneys and to protect the effects of haemorrhage.

Iron deficiency
The most common type of anaemia of pregnancy is due to iron de-

ficiency. The dietary intake of iron may be insufficient to meet the demands of both the mother and her child. She has increased her blood volume by 30 per cent to deal with all her own circulatory commitments, whilst the foetus requires iron for his own haemopoiesis as well as for storage in his liver in preparation for his scanty intake of iron during the first three months or so of life. In addition, absorption of iron from the gut may be defective, so that even if iron supplements are given they pass uselessly through the alimentary tract. Thirdly, the women most often in need of supplementary iron, often grande multiparae of low social class, are frequently irresponsible as regards their medication and fail to take their iron. For these reasons, a careful watch on haemoglobin levels must be maintained throughout pregnancy, and a minimum level of 80 per cent aimed for. Where the level is falling away, parenteral iron may be helpful and may be given as total dose iron dextran by intravenous drip. In such cases, the dose is calculated in terms of the patient's weight and haemoglobin deficit, according to charts prepared by the makers. This dose is added to 5 per cent dextrose solution, and run in at first very slowly because of the risk of anaphylactic reaction. This however is fortunately rare. The haemoglobin figure should rise by about one per cent per day, so that some time is required for a full response. If time is short and labour imminent, blood transfusion will be preferable.

Megaloblastic anaemia

A second type of anaemia seen in pregnancy is megaloblastic anaemia due to deficiency of folic acid, which interferes with the maturation of red cells. This anaemia may present rather acutely during the later weeks of pregnancy and as its name indicates, large immature nucleated red cells, megaloblasts, may be found in the peripheral blood or in the bone marrow. This is a hyperchromic anaemia, the reduced number of large red cells being well filled with haemoglobin, in contrast to the small hypochromic cells of iron deficiency anaemia. After the study of blood and marrow films to establish the diagnosis, transfusion may well be required. Subsequently treatment with iron and with folic acid in the therapeutic dosage of 5 mg thrice daily should be maintained until the pregnancy is over and even in the early weeks of the puerperium. Prophylactic treatment with iron and with folic acid in a lower dose of 300 mcg daily is valuable, but only if the patient takes the medication regularly.

In immigrant patients both from Asia, from Africa and from the shores of the Mediterranean, anaemia due to haemoglobinopathies, sickle cell anaemia and thalassaemia may be encountered; these will require skilled haematological investigation and treatment, but are rarely found in the indigenous population.

21

The use of drugs in pregnancy

Before any drug is given to a pregnant woman one must ask whether it may be teratogenic and liable to cause harm or abnormal development to the growing embryo. This is a very difficult problem, especially as the results of clinical trials in animals cannot with any certainty be extrapolated to man. For this reason there is very properly a tendency to extreme conservatism in the use of drugs in pregnancy, and they should be avoided if possible especially during the period of organogenesis, i.e. roughly the first trimester. At this time, treatment may be required for excessive vomiting, constipation and insomnia; there is a range of well-tried drugs available here including the phenobarbitones, promethazine theoclate (Avomine) or dicyclomine hydrochloride (Debendox) for sickness, relatively inert laxatives such as psyllium (Isogel) and long-used sedatives such as amyobarbitone which have never been incriminated as teratogens.

In certain cases of recurrent abortion, some obstetricians favour the use of progestogens, and here the nor-steroids such as norethisterone may cause virilization of a female foetus. The 17-α hydroxy-progesterones which have almost no androgenic properties will avoid this.

For the relief of pain in labour, pethidine and morphine are commonly used, and may cause respiratory depression in the foetus. This may be reversed with n-allyl normorphine (Lethidrone) or levallorphan (Lorfan) 0·5–1·0 mg given to the infant if he fails to breathe.

Oxytocic drugs may be used for the induction or stimulation of labour or to produce prolonged contraction of the uterus in order to prevent haemorrhage in the third or fourth stage of labour. Oxytocin, natural or synthetic, may be used for the former purpose, the dosage being adjusted according to the uterine response (Chapter 11). It produces short-lived contraction followed by relaxation as in normal labour, in contrast to the other commonly used oxytocic, ergometrine, which produces long-lasting tonic contraction. The action of oxytocin is obviously the more suited for induction of labour. There is no place for ergometrine before the birth of the child. In the third stage, however, the tonic contraction which it induces is just what is needed. Unfortunately ergometrine even if injected intra-muscularly is slow to act, and so Syntometrine, a combination of oxytocin and ergometrine is widely preferred. This gives the benefit of the rapid if transient action of oxytocin together with the slower but more prolonged action of ergometrine.

To effect uterine relaxation and relief of spasm, amyl nitrite by inhalation is effective but its action is transient. Isoxsuprine (Duvadilan) may be given by intravenous drip—this is somewhat unpredictable but its action when effective is prolonged. Diazepam (Valium) has also been recommended having been shown in vitro to produce myometrial relaxation, but its effectiveness is variable.

Antibiotics may be used for infections as in the non-pregnant but tetracycline is better avoided as it may lead to discolouration of the teeth of the infant. Sulphonamides should be used with caution, as the immature foetal liver may have difficulty in detoxicating them.

Many women today are on corticosteroids for asthma, rheumatic diseases and other complaints, and during pregnancy this may enhance any tendency to water retention due to toxaemia. For this reason the dosage should be kept as low as possible during pregnancy, but adequate cover with hydrocortisone should be provided during labour. This high dosage should be reduced as rapidly as possible, especially if operative delivery has been required, since it may adversely affect wound healing.

22

Family planning

There is an increasing concern throughout the world today about the control of population, since human fertility threatens to outrun world resources of food, water and space. On the individual level also, excessive fertility may be a problem and few can quarrel with the excellent slogan 'Every child a wanted child'. It is appropriate therefore that doctors and midwives who have responsibility for the care of pregnancies should also be able to advise their patients about family spacing and limitation.

METHODS OF CONTRACEPTION

Most methods of contraception are concerned with preventing the conjunction of the ovum and the sperm, and the efficiency of different methods varies. It is estimated that in every 100 couples of reproductive age having unprotected intercourse, 14 pregnancies per year will result.

The safe period

If intercourse is restricted to the safe period, i.e. to a time when no ovum is available for fertilization, and avoided completely from days 10–17 of a 28-day cycle, the rate of pregnancy will be around 7 per 100 women per year. This is the only method of contraception, apart from *complete abstinence* from intercourse, approved by the Roman Catholic Church. Its failures are largely due to the complete unpredictability of ovulation in any woman with an irregular cycle.

Coitus interruptus

Coitus interruptus, or withdrawal, when the male withdraws the

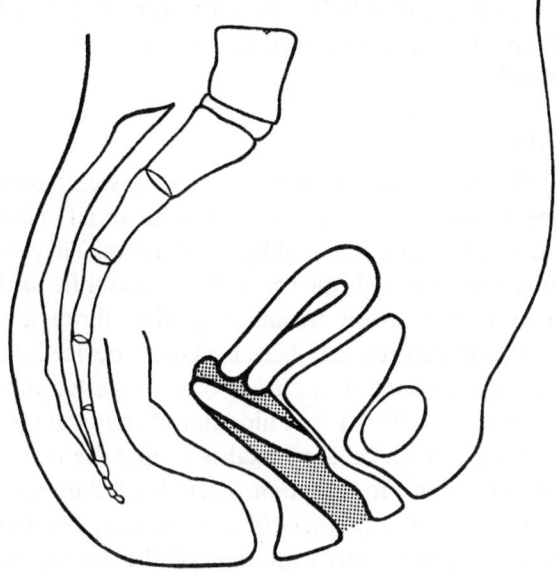

Fig.37. Contraceptive diaphragm in situ.

penis from the vagina before ejaculation, gives a similar failure rate and may be a cause of much frustration and many psychosomatic symptoms in both husband and wife, and of much marital disharmony, since the wife frequently fails to achieve orgasm.

Vaginal diaphragm

The occlusive methods include the vaginal diaphragm or Dutch cap (Fig.37) which must be inserted before intercourse to form a barrier across the upper vagina, from the upper margin of the symphysis to the posterior fornix, so as to exclude the sperm from the cervical canal.

The sheath

A similar method for the use of the male is the sheath, condom or French letter which is placed over the penis before intercourse, and this too is intended to prevent sperm reaching the cervix.

Spermicidal jellies

A variety of spermicidal jellies, creams, pessaries and foams are intended to destroy the sperms before they can enter the cervical canal. All of these methods carry a failure rate of about 3 pregnancies per 100 women/years (per 100 couples per year). When occlusive and spermicidal methods are combined, contraceptive efficiency is markedly increased.

The I.U.C.D.

The I.U.C.D. (or intra-uterine contraceptive devices) are of various shapes—loops, coils or spirals of plastic material usually radio-opaque and in some instances mildly radio-active. They are inserted with an introducer through the cervical canal, and lie in the uterine cavity, often with a nylon thread projecting through the cervix so that the wearer can reassure herself that the device is still in situ. Its mode of action is not clear; it has been suggested that it causes a low-grade endometritis so that nidation of the ovum is hindered, or that it interferes with tubal peristalsis so that the ovum does not reach the uterus in time for nidation. There is a failure rate here with the device in situ of 1·3–2·0 per 100 women/year, but there is also the problem of spontaneous expulsion of the device, and uterine cramps and menorrhagia in about 10 per cent of women may lead to demands for its removal. Its great advantage in women who tolerate it well is that no action is required 'on the night'.

Oral contraceptives

The combined oral contraceptives, 'the Pills', contain a progestogen with an oestrogen, and have virtually no failure rate if taken regularly. They do however demand conscientious self-medication by the patient. Most 'pills' today contain 0·5–1·0 mg of progestogen together with 50 mcg of an oestrogen, and are taken daily for 21 days from the 5th day of the cycle. Some preparations have seven dummy or placebo pills and are taken every day. The principal action of the 'pill' is to suppress ovulation, probably by inhibition of pituitary gonadotrophins, but a secondary action in making the cervical mucus hostile to the sperm is also probable. Most women tolerate them well, but there is no doubt that undesirable and even dangerous side-effects may occur in some women. The best known is an increased tendency to thrombo-embolic disease, commonly in the leg veins, but cerebral thrombosis has also been recorded. Changes in lipoid metabolism and in thyroid activity have been reported, and precipitation of a diabetic tendency is also recognized. In a few women, especially in Scandinavia a special type of cholestatic jaundice has been recorded. The 'pill' therefore should be avoided in women with a history of thrombo-embolism or with severe varicose veins which may predispose to this, and in those with abnormal thyroid function and abnormal lipid or carbohydrate metabolism. On the other hand, in the great majority of women the 'pill' is not only a safe and effective method of contraception, but it may produce positive benefits in improved control of menstruation. Jeffcoate has stated that the risk of death for the average woman using the pill is about the same as that from taking the car to the station to meet her husband each evening. Certainly the risks are in general much less than those of pregnancy and although the 'pill' is far from being the ideal contraceptive, it is at present probably the nearest approach to this available.

The 'sequential' pill, using oestrogen in the first half of the cycle and oestrogen and progestogen in the second half, although more closely mimicking the normal hormonal pattern, is less successful, and has a failure rate of about one per 100 women/years.

Continuous daily progestogens have also produced a similar failure rate, and control of the menstrual cycle has been poor. The incidence of thrombo-embolism however has been greatly reduced as compared with the combined tablets. The method was withdrawn because of the production of breast tumours in beagle bitches, but these are not malignant and it is doubtful if a similar risk exists in humans.

Depot injection. In order to overcome the necessity for regular medication the use of a depot injection of a progestogen every three months has been advocated. This however has carried a certain failure rate with poor cycle control, and has not gained wide acceptance.

Prostaglandin pill. A variety of 'morning after' pills has been advised, but none has proved widely acceptable. It may be that a prostaglandin pill, which will act as an abortifacient rather than a contraceptive, will be available in the near future, and may supply the 'do-it-yourself' facility which many desire.

Abortion
Abortion as a method of fertility control has been extensively used in Japan, where the birth-rate has been reduced so that population increase has been stabilized, but only at the cost of more abortions than live births. This method has also been used extensively in

Eastern Europe, but has never become widely popular, and is repugnant to most workers in this country. Prevention of pregnancy is regarded as a much better solution, and the policy of 'abortion on demand' has gained only limited acceptance in the United Kingdom.

Sterilisation

Sterilisation is commonly effected by interruption of the tubes, and one of the most popular and effective methods is Pomeroy's operation, whereby the middle thirds of the tubes are resected to prevent conjunction of ovum and sperm. Failure is rare, but occasional fallacies are the 'sterilization' of a round ligament and the failure to observe the very occasional presence of a third tube. The great objection to sterilisation is its irreversibility; operations to restore continuity of the tubes are possible, but the results in terms of successful pregnancy are so poor that one must warn one's patient, before she decides to be sterilised, that she must be prepared to abandon all hope of further children. Despite this, sterilisation is widely accepted by women with two, three or more children, and especially in women over 30 years of age who may have used other forms of contraception for some years.

Sterilisation may be carried out as an interval operation, but there are advantages in puerperal sterilisation carried out usually 24–48 hours after delivery. The mother is already in hospital, the tubes pushed up by the large puerperal uterus are easily accessible close to the anterior abdominal wall, and one can be confident that the woman is not pregnant. The operation should be planned long before, probably early in the pregnancy, and snap decisions are to be deplored. The matter should be discussed with husband and wife, and the husband may opt for vasectomy, best carried out during the wife's pregnancy. It is not unduly cynical however to remember that vasectomy of the husband does not necessarily mean that the wife will not become pregnant in our present permissive society.

In women with menstrual disorders, sterilisation by hysterectomy is becoming increasingly popular. In a woman whose cycle control is dependent upon her oral contraceptive, sterilisation will remove this support from her, and hysterectomy is obviously the method to be preferred.

Many of the unwanted babies in our society are born to women of low intelligence and low social class, whose failure to undertake contraception is largely due to irresponsibility. These women may be more responsibly motivated in the puerperium than at any other time, and the advice in this field of a trusted midwife may be acceptable and may be heeded to a greater degree than can be achieved from any other source. The importance therefore of a good understanding by the midwife of the general principles of family planning cannot be over-emphasized.

23

Vital statistics, maternal and foetal mortality

The vital statistics in any community reflect not only the quality of medical and nursing care, but also its nutritional and environmental state. World comparisons will usually show that the most advanced nations can produce the most favourable figures; on the other hand, the activities of such agencies as the World Health Organization have produced the most striking improvements in some of the most primitive countries, and paradoxically this has in many cases led to a worsening of problems of overpopulation and consequent malnutrition.

Within any one community, the vital statistics can be used as a yardstick of social and medical progress, and in obstetrics, the mortality results for mother and child have given some cause for satisfaction in that they have shown progressive improvement over the past 70 years. *The death rate* (number of deaths per 1000 total population) has fallen faster than the *birth rate* (number of births per 1000 total population) with a consequent progressive increase in population. In 1901, the death rate was 16·9, in 1965 it was 11·5, whilst the birth rate, 28·7 in 1901, has fluctuated during the past 10 years between 18·2 in 1963 and 16·0 in 1970. Considerations of these figures will indicate the disparity between birth and death rates and vital importance of the measures discussed in the previous chapter.

MATERNAL MORTALITY RATE

The maternal mortality rate (number of maternal deaths per 1000 births) has fallen progressively from 4·27 in 1901 to 0·24 in 1969. This gratifying result reflects the work of public health authorities, nutritionists and economists as well as doctors and midwives, but it is salutary to reflect that the triennial report of the Confidential Enquiry into Maternal Deaths published by the Ministry of Health invariably finds that avoidable factors were present in around half the cases. The blame may rest upon the patient herself—only a few women nowadays have no ante-natal care and fewer still lack skilled attention in labour, but defaulters from clinics may place themselves at risk; this is particularly true of the over-burdened grande multipara of poor intelligence and low social class, a group which makes a disproportionate contribution to the mortality statistics. In some cases the blame must lie upon the medical and nursing attendants, and errors of judgement, as for example in the choice of place of confinement or neglect of regular observation of haemoglobin or blood-pressure levels, may set the scene for subsequent death of the mother.

Causes

The causes of maternal deaths have altered over the years, and haemorrhage and sepsis, formerly the great killers, have been to some extent controlled by better nutrition, with improved resistance both to blood loss and to infection, and increased availability of blood banks and powerful anti-infective agents. In this advance the great increase in hospital confinement, bringing the patient within easy reach of all the facilities needed for her treatment, has played a large part.

Anaesthetic deaths. In recent years, anaesthetic deaths have become a leading cause of maternal mortality, and the problems presented and the measures available to solve them have been discussed in Chapter 16.

Pulmonary embolism. Another great cause of death is pulmonary embolism, which may occur acutely and without warning. It has recently been shown that the clinical diagnosis of thrombo-phlebitis is grossly inaccurate and that radio-active scanning methods will show mis-diagnosis in up to 50 per cent of cases. A number of research projects are in progress endeavouring both to improve diagnosis and to prevent thrombo-phlebitis. Automatic massage of the limbs in the puerperal or post-operative patient with a pulsed inflatable cuff has recently given good results, and the intravenous administration of low molecular weight dextran is claimed to prevent sludging of blood platelets and so to be a valuable prophylactic. In the average patient however one must still rely on such measures as are described in Chapter 7, avoidance of anaemia and trauma, leg movements and early ambulation.

Cardiac disease. A third great cause of maternal death today is cardiac disease, and despite advances in both medical and surgical management of the diseases of the heart, the most valuable method of combating this problem is probably the prevention of pregnancy in the severely affected individual. The liberal use of sterilisation in this group will pay dividends.

Toxaemia and its complications still claim their victims, usually from renal failure or cerebro-vascular accidents, but with proper ante-natal care and judicious management these should be fewer.

Haemorrhage and sepsis are still responsible for many deaths, often following abortion, but also in later pregnancy especially in neglected cases. The effect upon illegal abortion of the 1968 Abortion Act is not yet clear, but a number of deaths have been reported where so-called therapeutic abortion has been carried out in unsuitable circumstances.

INFANT MORTALITY RATE

The other aspect of the work of the obstetrician and midwife is reflected in the vital statistics for the infant.

The stillbirth rate (the number of deaths per 1000 live and still-births) indicates the number of infants 'who born after the 28th week of pregnancy and after complete expulsion from the mother, neither breathe nor show any other sign of life'. These deaths are due to a variety of causes, including placental failure due usually to toxaemia or to constitutional causes (Chapter 19), hydrops foetalis from rhesus sensitization (Chapter 17), cord accidents, syphilis, dominance of a larger twin etc. In such cases, the foetus may have been dead for some time, and will be found at birth to be macerated, with the epidermis peeling off. In other cases, the stillbirth is due to birth trauma and is due usually to intra-cranial haemorrhage (Chapter 19) resulting from precipitate delivery, excessive moulding or trauma from instrumental or breech delivery.

The early neonatal mortality rate (deaths in the first week of life per 1000 live births) gives a better idea of the work of obstetric units than do the neonatal mortality and infant mortality rates which deal with deaths in the first month and the first year respectively, since these latter rates reflect the effect of intercurrent disease and accidents, whereas the early neonatal mortality is due largely to abnormalities arising during pregnancy.

The perinatal mortality rate. The total of stillbirths and first week neonatal deaths is expressed as the perinatal mortality rate per 1000 live and stillbirths, and this is perhaps the best measure of the success of one's management of the pregnancies under one's care. The perinatal mortality in England and Wales has fallen from 38·5 in 1948 to 23·0 in 1970, a less striking improvement than that shown in maternal mortality which fell by almost 80 per cent during the same period but none the less a progressive advance, with the 1970 figures the lowest ever recorded. The principal causes of early neonatal death include prematurity, with respiratory distress syndrome frequently the immediate cause of death, intra-cranial haemorrhage, trauma, congenital deformity and haemolytic disease all of which have been discussed in Chapters 16, 17 and 19.

The Perinatal Mortality Survey of 1958 pointed the way to improvements in all these figures, and many of the conclusions to be drawn from it have already been reflected in improved management and more acceptable mortality rates. It is to be hoped that a further survey which is in prospect now will confirm that some of the errors found in 1958 have now been eliminated, and that it will indicate the ways in which still further improvement may be possible.

Index

dystocia
   cervical   103
   shoulder   15

Early neonatal mortality rate   153
eclampsia   93, 94
   diagnosis of   95
   treatment of   94
EDD (estimated date of delivery)
   35, 98
endocrine control of pregnancy   22
endometrium   21, 23
epidural block   117
episiotomy   48, 115
essential hypertension   96
examination
   general   37
   of blood   37
   of foetus   92
   of pelvis   40
   of urine   36
external cephalic version   70
external female genitalia   13

Face presentation   73
family planning   144
Fallopian tubes   10
female pelvis   61
fertilisation   26
fertilised ovum   26
   development of   26
fibrinolysis   80
foetal distress   107
foetal heart rate   107
foetal movement   107
foetal skull   15
foetus (examination of)   92
foetus papyraceus   60
forewaters   45, 98, 121
FSH (follicle-stimulating hormone)
   19
FSHRH (follicle-stimulating
   hormone releasing hormone)   19
fundal height   38, 39
funic presentation   99

General examination   37
generally contracted pelvis   61
genes   24, 119
glycosuria   37
gonorrhoea   124
Graafian follicle   20
grande multipara   51, 87
gynaecoid pelvis   61

Haemolytic disease   119
haemorrhage   152
   accidental   78
   ante-partum   78
   intra-cranial   16, 132
   post-partum   83, 86
hip-bone (innominate)   3
hydatidiform mole   38, 88
hydramnios   56, 137
hydrocephalus   135
hydrops foetalis   120
   treatment of   121
hyperemesis gravidarum   35
hypertonicity of uterus   105
hypofibrinogenaemia   80
hypoglycaemia   131
hypotensive agents   91
hypothalamus   22
hysterectomy   87, 148

Incoordinate uterine action   103
   causes of   105
   management of   104
induction of labour   97
   indications for   97
   methods of   98
   medical induction   100
   surgical induction   99
infant mortality rate   152
infection (urinary)   14, 53
injuries (at birth)   132
innominate bone   3, 4
internal version   76
intervention in labour   109
intra-cranial haemorrhage   16, 132
IUCD (intra-uterine contraceptive
   device)   146
intra-uterine death   137
investigations
   radiological   32
   routine   36
iron deficiency   139

Kidneys   13
Kielland's forceps   112
Kleihauer-Betke technique   122
Kochers' forceps   112

Labour   42, 58
   onset of   43
   first stage of   45
   second stage of   46
   third stage of   46
   induction of   97